# *JOURNEY TO JOY*

*An Inspirational Memoir*

Joy Walker

Published by BookLocker.com, Inc., St. Petersburg, Florida.

Printed on acid-free paper.

BookLocker.com, Inc.
2016

# Dedication

To Daddy and Mama, in gratitude for their legacy of faith. To my siblings and their offspring; to my children and my descendants yet unborn. To the glory of God.

"You brought me out of the womb; you made me trust in you, even at my mother's breast. From birth I was cast on you; from my mother's womb you have been my God." Psalm 22:9, 10

# Table of Contents

# FOREWORD

"In *Journey to Joy*, the author traverses life like a true woman of faith. A masterful writer and storyteller with a wise and open heart, she embraces life to the fullest...the good, bad and ugly. Joy so passionately and reflectively emotes through the written word that her writing comes to life and seems to escape the confines of the pages.

Joy tells of her breast cancer experience, recounting her journey from patient to advocate for herself and others. She engagingly describes her blossoming to survivor and even thriver! This is a must read for patients, survivors, family members and caregivers.

Anyone who has lived through divorce and single parenting will find validation in the author's candid depiction of the insecurities and hurts common to these struggles. The reader will be moved and affirmed as she demonstrates that even our most painful trials can be surmounted when we can hold on to purpose and joy. Every parent, single or not, can derive inspiration and hope. Through her tears and laughter, between the lines, there is always *Joy*. Her pursuit of ultimate fulfillment through her faith will certainly inspire yours. What a gift she has courageously and creatively given!"—*Kimlin Tam Ashing, Ph.D.; Professor, Beckman Research Institute; Founding Director, CCARE (Center of Community Alliance for Research & Education), City of Hope Medical Center*

# ABOUT THE AUTHOR

"Over the past few years, Joy has struggled, seeking to know and understand her purpose in life. But as far back as I can remember, and to this very day, she has somehow managed to be continuously purposeful in the life she lives, the gifts she gives and the way she loves and serves. Whether she is actively inspiring others through her poetry and music, offering encouragement or admonition by sharing lessons learned from personal experiences, giving targeted gifts that meet the need of the moment, or pouring her creative energies into homeschooling her children, Joy has been a life-building force to those around her.

On a more personal note, my big sister, Joy has been my unwitting mentor. I have learned valuable life lessons by literally sitting at her feet. As a child, I helped Joy count and sort the money she earned by selling her handmade crafts. She accounted for every penny. Despite her own lack, she would not only set aside funds for her tithe to the church, but would designate another portion to sponsor a child living in poverty, or to bless someone else in need. That non-verbal life lesson has gone a long way. After watching Joy courageously navigate her way through life with a Braille book in one hand and a cane in the other, I knew, when my turn came, that I would be able to navigate my way through legal blindness as well.

Joy is an inspirer. She has purposefully taken the time to document her journey. The life lessons learned, as recounted in *Journey to Joy,* encourage others to forge their way through life's difficulties towards the joy that comes in discovering their purpose. There is no greater accomplishment than to leave a positive imprint on the spirit of another human being?"—*Faith Walker Marshall*

# PREFACE

*Journey to Joy* is a treasury of poems, essays, letters, and journal entries, chronicling the author's journey from a shy teenager saddled with the shocking news of potential blindness to a 68-year-old senior with congestive heart failure. Her album of memories transports the reader through years of struggle in establishing her identity and purpose. She describes her arduous trek to a B.A. degree, a tumultuous marriage and divorce, the drama and trauma of single parenting, breast cancer, bereavement and more.

Her pilgrimage, gut-wrenching yet sprinkled with humor, ultimately leads to the triumph of faith and joy as the author learns to trust in God's sufficient grace.

"Consider it pure joy, my friends, whenever you face trials of many kinds, because you know that the testing of your faith develops perseverance. Perseverance must finish its work so that you may be mature and complete, not lacking anything." James 1:2-4

# ACKNOWLEDGEMENTS

The creation of this book was providential from start to finish. I am overwhelmed at God's extravagant provision of people and means. Becky and Pete Meyers, thank you for the practical demonstration of your belief in me. Thanks to my church family for help with the computer upgrade as I began, and for your prayerful support.

Thanks to Candice and Jonathan Pulos and Bob and Sue Sweetman, my trusted computer techies. Wajida Alhambra, you saved me from dumping much of the content of this book. Thanks also for the laser printer from your garage, donated just as my ink-jet printer died. Faith Marshall and Carol Walker, my beloved sisters, thanks for your constant encouragement and prayers; you were there when I wanted to tear my hair out. Carol, you kept reminding me that I had already "written a library" and just needed to organize my material. You were so right!

For hours of meticulous editing, thanks to Anne Oshita, George Fawrup, Daniel Vera, Diana Gegala, Gloria Rios, Sam Kim, Joan Smith, Linda Ghabril, Janet Ervin, and Candace Nicholson. You rescued me from the monotony of my screen reader. The emotions expressed as you read helped give life to the manuscript and gave me feedback on its impact. Thank you Adrienne Min for hours of brainstorming about the book cover, helping me visualize the end product. Mark Christiansen and David Oswald, your expertise with the photos was invaluable.

Jeanne Lawrence, Julie Davey, Chris Gonzalez and Kimlin Ashing, I appreciate your favorable endorsement of the book. I could never have accomplished this feat without each of you. Above all, I thank God for the gifts He has given and the opportunities to use them.

# INTRODUCTION

In this compendium of poetry and prose, I paint a panoramic view of my quest for identity and meaning. There have been many unfathomable questions on the journey. As I struggled from trials (through lessons gleaned from failure) to triumphs, I had to humbly acknowledge that God is God, and I am not. Some things are beyond my understanding, but my faith in Jesus always brings me back from defeat and failure to renewed joy and purposeful living.

William Wordsworth defines poetry as "...the spontaneous overflow of powerful feelings: it takes its origin from emotion recollected in tranquility." I am a deep thinker, and writing poetry has proved cathartic in my attempts to unravel life's riddles. Some poems were conceived in my deepest pain and were indeed the unplanned outbursts of emotions. Others were born after arduous labor, providing answers to life's perplexities or reminding me of truths forgotten in the turmoil.

Although I was named Joy, it has taken many years and many trials to appreciate the full meaning of my name. When confronted with problems, at first I tend to see the glass as half empty and must work at accepting it as half full. On this journey, I have found that a sense of humor is a necessity. If I cannot laugh at myself and my predicament, I cannot survive.

Someone once said, "If only you hadn't lost your sight, you could have done so much more!" She was comparing me with classmates who had become "successful" according to cultural norms. Did she assume that my value is derived from social status or scholarship? My life's value is not measured by possessions, fortune or fame (Luke 12:15). I am uniquely designed and gifted by God, limitations and all. My role is to accomplish my God-assigned purpose, no more and no less. My job is to flourish in my designated sphere of influence. I have worn many hats and played various roles, though not always applauded. I have been a wife, mother, domestic engineer, nurse, nutritionist, financial advisor, home teacher, counselor, poet, musician and friend. Need I say more?

5

A "liberated" woman once made the disparaging remark that anyone with a college degree who becomes a stay-at-home mom is like one carrying a "pearl in the apron pocket." Well, a pearl is still a pearl no matter where you keep it; besides, I added two more pearls to that one, and those gems never depreciate. The most productive and fulfilling years of my life were spent raising two beautiful children, my gifts to the world.

Raising children is a challenge. Raising children as a single parent is a bigger challenge. Raising children as a legally blind single parent is a gargantuan challenge. Oh, and let's not forget about raising hormonal teenagers as a menopausal legally blind single parent with cancer. The first chemo treatment threw me into a medically-induced menopause, the worst kind. It was in rising to face those challenges that I discovered irreplaceable joy.

At the end of my senior year in college, the dorm director gifted me with a poster that said: "To achieve all that is possible, we must attempt the impossible. To be all that we can be, we must dream to be more" (John C. Maxwell). That is how I have tried to live. When I felt the call to homeschool my children, I had no idea how it would happen. However, God, who qualifies the called rather than calling the qualified, steered me through that process. It was a "road less traveled," and I had many critics who have, in time, changed their tune. Not that it mattered; I knew I had chosen the right path.

When my husband of 11 years defected, I was devastated. In my grief and soul-searching, I realized the mistake I had made. I had assumed he would fulfill my joy. As painful as it was to admit, his leaving forced me to refocus in the right direction. God is the source of my joy, and I had lost track of that truth.

Marriage is, at best, a union of two broken, imperfect people. The search for joy is fruitless until each one recognizes and surrenders to the truth that "My soul finds rest in God alone..." (Psalm 62:1). Though for a season I doubted God's love for me, I have seen His faithfulness displayed in ways I would never have known without the heartache of divorce. There have been countless opportunities to experience His presence and provision. I am now single and satisfied because Jesus supplies all that I lack. When I am weak, He gives me strength; when I am sad, He gives me joy. He also sends loving friends to bolster me in times of need.

In the past, I would panic when a trusted friend or helper needed to move on. Being legally blind, I must depend on others. I have an independent spirit, but I am not foolish. I have had to acknowledge the liabilities presented by my disability and ask for help where necessary. It's the only way to live successfully. While depending on others, I must remember that my ultimate dependence is on God. He promises to meet my needs (Philippians 4:19). Now, when a helper is no longer available, instead of panicking, I remind myself that God is my source and will keep His promise. He has never failed me.

Cancer brought the reality of my mortality to the forefront. Immersed in the agony of rejection, I wasn't sure I wanted to go on. Discovery of the lump catapulted me into action. If I really wanted to die, all I had to do was nothing. Of course, I couldn't give up. My children needed me.

The mammogram was sandwiched between two days in court. First, the children and I met with their father and a mediator to settle visitation and financial issues. The following day, a mammogram confirmed the lump; a biopsy was ordered. A day later, the judge discussed my visual impairment and asked if I had any other physical problems. I said no; I wanted the lump to be benign.

Knowing my days were numbered, how would I spend them? It was not my time to go, but how would I live until then? I realized that, even in my woundedness, whether from a failed marriage or from cancer, I could bring joy to others who were hurting. Staying wrapped up in my pain brought me no gain. Jesus Himself is a wounded healer and called me to be likewise.

There is no pretending in this book. I express love, hope, disappointment, anger, compassion, pain, anguish, fear, faith, humor, forgiveness, and ultimately joy. Women often open their hearts in candid response to the sentiments expressed in my poetry, confirming the universality of the struggle. Some poems reflect the stories of women who often voiced their appreciation for my precise portrayal of feelings they were unable to verbalize.

To women or men who are hurting, I pray that this book will call you out of denial to face your fears. Find deliverance in a God who loves you and wants you whole. Recognize your value in God's eyes, and do not allow anyone to discount that value. Seek Him as the source of your joy. Let God fill your cup so you can give out of the abundant overflow of His love. True liberation comes from Jesus, who longs to complete your joy.

Life is difficult at best; I will not pretend otherwise; but I have choices. I can live in debilitating denial or courageously embrace reality, however harsh. I can extend forgiveness to those who hurt me or let the acid of bitterness corrode my heart. I can choose to profit from pain or play the blame game. I can flog myself for past failures or forgive my human frailty. I can turn my back on God or seek His strength to see me through. I can choose to devalue myself, as others have, or accept the unconditional love that Jesus offers me. I can choose defeat or joy. I choose joy!

"You have made known to me the path of life; you will fill me with joy in your presence, with eternal pleasure at your right hand." Psalm 16:11

# PART 1. EARLY CHALLENGES

## BUMPS IN THE ROAD

Halfway across Maxfield Avenue, I suddenly heard the roar of a motorbike barreling toward Paul and me. By the time the bike and its rider entered my field of vision, it was too late. I panicked. My next sensation was slowly waking to darkness, hearing an excited crowd and the ambulance siren.

My brother and I had been on our way to Friday evening youth group. He made it across safely and ran back home to alert the family. Our terrified parents accompanied me in the ambulance. Because the focus was on my complaint of a severe headache, my fractured left knee was not discovered until the next morning. That summer was spent in a full leg cast, and I still have scars on my lower leg from the battering and bruising it received. I was 16.

During the elementary school years, my family lived in a tenement house that faced the back of the dormitories belonging to the Salvation Army School for the Blind. As my siblings and I played in the front yard, students often called to us through the wooden window blinds. My sister, Grace, Paul and I attended the elementary school a few yards from home and adjacent to the school for the blind. The trash outside the blind school stirred our curiosity. There were papers and whole books covered in bumps. We played with the papers, rubbing our fingers over the bumps, ignorant of their significance.

In 1960, passing the Common Entrance Exam, Grace and I won scholarships to an all-girls high school in Kingston. A secondary education was not free, so this called for great celebration in our family. Two years later, Jamaica won her independence from British colonial rule. There was much festivity as people celebrated with merrymaking and dancing in the streets. We proudly sang our national anthem, as the Union Jack was lowered and Jamaica's flag of black, green and gold was raised.

9

As a young girl, I loved reading but began to seriously struggle in high school. I had difficulty reading the fine print of language dictionaries used in my Spanish and Latin classes. Math was a challenge as numbers were often distorted. Reading the comic strips in the newspaper had been a favorite pastime, until that became difficult too. I usually sat in the front row in order to see the chalkboard and didn't enjoy playing games that involved catching a ball. "Butterfingers" was my name on the netball court. No one wanted me on their team. After being hit in the face by the ball, I would put my hands up to protect myself, never sure where the ball was coming from or where it would land.

Because my vision was decreasing gradually rather than suddenly, I don't think my parents fully understood the trauma. Daddy said I was making myself miserable; besides, they couldn't afford a doctor. An affluent relative soon heard about the problem and offered to pay for a visit to the optician. At the age of 15, I started wearing glasses, but soon realized they didn't make much difference. As an adolescent, I was already challenged with establishing my self-identity, and this new dilemma did not help.

An ophthalmologist directed me to read the eye chart, I asked, "What chart?" I slowly moved my head around trying to locate it. At the University Hospital, doctors and interns took turns peering into my eyes while mouthing their fascination. A social worker told me to hurry up and do whatever I wanted to do with my life; I was going to be blind. Alone when this thunderbolt struck, I sat in stunned silence.

Already an introvert and never part of the popular crowd, I was embarrassed when asked to read my essay to the class. Unable to decipher my own handwriting, I stuttered like a bumbling fool. In chemistry lab, the students giggled when the teacher called me "clumsy." I was waving the test tube next to the Bunsen burner instead of directly over the flame. Sauntering toward the bus terminal after school, girls would fall back a few paces just to watch me "kiss" the light post. I laughed with them, but actually felt like an idiot.

At home, I bumped into furniture; on the street, I walked into parked cars and collided with people head on. Neighbors accused me of being a snob when I failed to recognize them, while strangers rescued me from approaching danger. Some friends doubted my veracity; others, oblivious to my inner turmoil, were convinced I was handling it well. They couldn't detect my faltering faith. I began relying on man, rather than on God, ultimately a disillusioning decision.

The following incident, amusing only in retrospect, confirmed my worsening vision.

## MANGO HARVEST

We lived at Berwick Road, #1B,
With heavy-laden mango trees.
When Daddy went to harvest some,
I said I'd help since I was home.

As Daddy lifted up the stick,
I cupped my hands to catch the pick.
I saw just one where Daddy aimed,
Had plum forgot my eyes were lame.

I saw just one, I am no dunce,
But three were hanging in a bunch.
Three mangoes came careening down
Upon my head then hit the ground;

Huge Haden mangoes, one, two, three,
With great precision fell on me.
Bang! Bam! Bop! Bash! Splat! Plop!
Then busted on the ground they plopped.

I saw just one, I tell the truth!
Soon I saw stars instead of fruit.
Grabbing my disbelieving head,
Crying and mangoless I went to bed.

Haile Selassie, Emperor of Ethiopia, created historical momentum upon his arrival in Jamaica on April 21$^{st}$, 1966. He was hailed by thousands of Rastafarians who deemed him their Messiah, a claim he denied. That was a significant year for me as well. Graduating from high school in June (after A level exams), I obtained an entry level position in a government office in Kingston. My success was short-lived. After two or so years, failing the medical portion of the civil service exam, I soon received a letter of dismissal. It was suggested I find another job that didn't require good vision.

The blow wasn't so much the loss of the job per se, but its implications. Something was wrong with me; I wasn't normal. By the time I became unemployed, my parents and five siblings had left the country. Being separated from my family for the first time in 21 years increased feelings of loneliness and depression.

When Mrs. Urquhart, a former elementary school teacher, heard of my dilemma, she sent me to Captain Lucaris at the School for the Blind. "Tell her you want to learn Braille." Initially, it was fun, like learning a new language, and soon I was reading and writing Braille. The bumps now made sense, and Captain Lucaris loaned me a Perkins Brailler for practice.

A year after my family had migrated to America, my mom's uncle, who resided in Boston, came home for a visit. Concerned about my depression, Uncle Boysie consulted a doctor at Massachusetts Eye and Ear Infirmary. He made an appointment and sent me the confirmation letter. This enabled me to obtain a one-year medical visa.

In 1970, Dr. Eliot Berson diagnosed me with paracentral retinitis pigmentosa with macular degeneration. This was a progressive, degenerative disease with a recessive genetic link. I was declared legally blind, having lost most of my central vision. After conducting a family study, Dr. Berson published a paper with my case history. Carol and Faith, two of my three sisters, received a similar diagnosis some years later. Before returning to Jamaica, I researched resources for vision impairment, and started the paperwork for my permanent visa.

Accepting my new reality, I resolved to acquire some new skills. A musician friend was developing a play-by-ear course and needed a test student. I had always desired to learn piano, but my parents couldn't afford lessons. He taught me the basics for a year. Having a natural ear for music, I applied myself, and before long, was playing for the youth group, church services and choir. I even taught myself to play the accordion.

Meanwhile, with the hope of finding a job, I learned to touch-type at a local evening school. The teacher was reluctant to make the necessary accommodations for me to develop proficiency with the Dictaphone. I couldn't hold a typing job without using this device, so I felt cheated. Learning macramé and Popsicle stick art, I developed my own designs and sold my creations to friends and neighbors. Under the auspices of the Jamaica Society for the Blind, I earned a small stipend teaching macramé to two older blind women.

On the last day of high school, I said goodbye to friends with short verses I composed. My poems were well received, and I discovered a gift. Having had only a modicum of training in writing poetry, I couldn't envision the major role this gift would play on my journey past life's bumps and thumps. The choir director at my church fostered my musical skills as well as my poetry writing. In 1972, he played a pivotal role in helping me publish *Memories*, my first book of poems. Proceeds from the sale paid for my return ticket to Boston.

As I disembarked at Logan Airport, a stranger pressed some money into my hand and hurried off the plane. I smiled to myself. Little did he know; that "poor blind girl" was richer than she had ever been. I had money in my pocket, earned from my own ingenuity.

## MIXED MEMORIES

As higher and higher up life's hill I climb,
Steeper and steeper the pathway I find,
And mixed are the memories lingering
Of people, places, moments and things.

Sweet are the memories that lighten my step,
That cause me to smile and my sorrows forget,
Of friends who have faithfully done their part
And secured a permanent place in my heart.

Some are still with me, others are gone,
But never, never will I forget one,
For moments of pleasure that I can recall
Are filled with faces of friends great and small.

Times when I've stumbled or miserably failed
Remind me that I'm only human and frail.
Yet even these memories serve to sustain
And strengthen for struggles that still remain.

More sobering still are the memories of grief
When adversity's whip made me cower and weep,
Yet in some reflections the pain distant seems
Like the shadowy sensations we get in dreams.

Some memories remain still poignant with pain,
Making me hurt and weep again.
Some I can share with my closest friends,
Some will be secret until life ends.

# *I SHALL MISS YOU ALL*

Now my friends, I've a story to tell.
I do hope you'll all enjoy it right well.
It's about a family of members ten.
I do hope this history won't dry my pen.
You may notice some variations in meter,
But variation is supposed to make life sweeter.

Daddy woke up one bright sunny morn
And searched his wallet as he gave a big yawn.
"Someone was in here! I miss some money!"
"How much, Daddy?" "Five shillings, Sonny."
"You said I could take it to buy me some sweets,
You told me so last night while you were asleep."

Mama, oh boy! She is such a narrator!
With a love for detail, who could be greater?
You could sit listening for almost an hour
Trying her foremost point to discover.
She is really telling you what John had said,
But first you must hear of her ancestors dead.

Now what is that I hear like a tread?
It must be Aunt Adah getting out of bed.
"Paul, Paul!" she shouts in a whisper,
"Come on home you crazy mister!
You mean its midnight and you're still out there?
It would never happen if I were here!"

Just because I have some trouble in seeing,
Paul asked, "You sweeping the floor or ceiling?"
Fuming with anger, I lowered my head,
But missed him and hit the wall instead.
"Ha, ha, ha!" He laughed in glee,
"Joy looked at the wall and thought it was me."

So you won't stop pulling down the place?
All right! This minute I'll send for Grace.
Now here she comes, the disciplinarian
Wearing mod earrings and a pair of red pants.
"Come here to me, you naughty brats!"
Now all is so peaceful. How is that?

Now Paul, he is quite a sad case,
Thinks he's the handsomest guy in the place.
No barber would live who depends on him,
For he thinks his hair too nice to be trimmed.
One day I searched it looking for fleas;
He cried out in anguish, "My curls, oh please!"

Where there is work, Carol is never about.
To get her to work you must give her a clout;
But anytime salt fish is around,
She's the sweetest girl in this part of town.
She will do anything just to get a big bite,
And if it comes to that, she will even fight.

"Who made that mess? Lord, please help us!"
"Daniel, Mama," they cried in chorus.
"Now who's that getting on like a lion?"
"Daniel; Paul hit him with a piece of iron."
Put that Daniel in a lion's cage
And he'd eat up the lion in his terrible rage.

Patrick, he makes the greatest inventions,
But for fibbing he hasn't found the prevention.
If a soldier's bullet could bounce off his toes,
What will happen next, only Heaven knows!
With a mind so vivid he should be using a pen,
They should be partners, himself and Ken.

Baby chicks shouldn't eat cockroaches,
At least this is what little Faith supposes.
"Those nasty things will make him catch germs,
He shouldn't even be eating worms!"
So to get the roach out she squeezed the chick's head,
And when she stopped squeezing, the poor chick was dead!

How much I shall miss you all—
Mama, Faith, Carol, Danny, Patrick and Paul.
I know I shall be feeling quite blue
When I look around and see none of you.
After so many years now off they go;
When I'll see them again, only Heaven knows! 1968


## WHY I WRITE POETRY

I'm a poet in my humble way,
How I came to be I cannot say.
The gift was simply given to me
By the Lord Almighty.
If of this talent I'm bereaved,
A void within me it would leave.
It courses through my very veins,
Without it I would be insane.

I thank the Lord for this great gift,
So oft' it gives my spirit a lift
And countless hours to me has brought
Of thrilling moments and thrilling thoughts.
I write what I see inside of me,
I write what no one else can see,
I'm at my best in solitude
When I've on my thoughts a long time chewed.

Sometimes, as if by the wave of a wand,
There's pen and paper in my hand,
And how the words flow easy and free,
Thrilling in their beauty!
The world may never appraise my work,
But I will never from it shirk.
I must obey the urge to write
Even in the dead of night.

When inspiration beckons me,
I follow her most willingly.
Such wondrous stories she repeats,
Of life, love, loss, and grace in grief.
And as she speaks with joy I flush.
Sometimes I can't write fast enough,
And when she's gone, her story told,
The treasure left is more than gold. 1969


## *REKINDLED FIRE*

Last night I had a dream
So sweet and so serene.
The dream is gone, but in my heart
Gleams a rekindled fire.

There in the land of dreams
Close by a tiny stream
We sat, his head upon my breast.
His breath revived the flames.

The silvery moonlight shone,
Its magic 'round us spun
A net of love that bound us close.
The flame it stronger grew.

We talked of days to come
When we would share a home,
When we, forever joined as one,
Would share our hearts' desires.

We then in sweet repose
Reclined, our eyelids closed.
O what a blessed peace was there
Amid loves burning fire.

It ended all too soon
This dream of joy and boon.
But still its pleasant memories
Are lingering with me.

Whatever can it mean
This hope-inspiring dream?
Does it foretell my destiny
In this rekindled fire?

## NIPPED IN THE BUD

I wandered through the garden,
Looked at my favorite tree.
Till now, all that it ever bore
Were prickles, all for me.

At last there was a rosebud;
My heart leaped at the sight!
I watered it with tender care
By day and even by night.

The presence of that rosebud
Did cheer a lonesome heart;
That heart too soon made glad
Is now by sorrow torn apart.

I hoped that my sweet rosebud
Would bloom into a rose.
To hope for such a miracle
Was too much, I suppose.

I visited my garden,
Went to my favorite tree,
Reached out to touch my rosebud,
But just prickles greeted me.

Maybe some happy morning
A bud will come to stay,
To grow, to bloom into a rose;
I long for such a day!

Is this too much to hope for?
Or should I contented be
To stare in lonesome longing
At the prickles on my tree?


## A BIRTHDAY MESSAGE

Never give up
Though the clouds are dark with storm clouds overhead.
Only look up!
'Neath the clouds you'll see a silver lining spread.
Even though it now seems drear,
Love will fill your heart with cheer.
So, my dear, brush away those tears,
Care will soon give place to laughter.

Only hope, never fear,
Time is hope's best friend, my daughter!


## A FRIEND INDEED

When the birds are singing and the sky is blue,
When the sun is shining I can find you.
When life's worth living and joys are new
And I am smiling, I can find you.
But when the birds are silent and the sky is dark,
When the raindrops splatter and the teardrops start,
When my heart is aching and I cannot see,
When life's a burden, then you find me. 1970


## TO WHOM IT MAY CONCERN

What nerve of you to think I'd cry
The vision out of my poor eye!
Do you suppose there are no more men
But you, for me to apprehend?
The thought that I should lose my sight
Just over you, appalls me quite!

Tell me, young man, do I look
Like some fool read of in your book?
Do you suppose that to elate
Your haughty self I would create
Emotional upheavals wild?
Come on! Do you think I'm still a child?

Do you suppose I'd fret all day
Or cry my heart out in dismay?
Oh no, I'd not so foolish be,
I'll boldly face reality.

I love you and you don't love me.
What can I do if that must be?

I really wish that I could help,
For help you need, my dear young whelp.
You're not even the cat's brassiere,
Much more his pajamas, dear!
You mustn't so conceited be
Or you'll end in tragedy. 1969


## TO REAL FRIENDS

Friendship is like a tree,
Its roots grow deeper with time;
Its shade provides a haven
Of rest on life's weary climb.
A friend is a priceless gift,
A needed one, for sure,
And the one who has no friend
Cannot be unhappy more.

The one who is near in joy,
Yet nearer in times of need,
The one who cares when you are sad,
I call her a friend indeed.
The one who admits when you're right
But says you are wrong without fear,
The one who tries to understand,
Such is a friend sincere.

Many say they're your friends,
And you may believe they are,
But it never takes very long
To prove who your real friends are.

Friends will quarrel at times,
Have misunderstandings, I know,
But misunderstandings cleared away
Make the friendship stronger grow.

The strength of a tree is not known
Till the storm has come and passed.
Only then can you know its worth,
If the tree withstood the blast.
So in light of all that I've said,
I thank God for friendship true,
And pray that I'll worthy be
Of the friendship I've found in you.


## SILENT SONG

I remember magical moments
When dreams were possible,
When Aspiration beckoned me from Heaven
Daring me to climb the clouds.
I reveled in daydreaming and sang a happy song.
Then clouds of another sort invaded my horizon,
Dark, ominous clouds, heavy with foreboding.
The storm broke, and lightning struck.
My balloon fizzled, and the singing stopped.
Having neither will nor skill to scale the walls
My new reality had erected,
I cringed before the task of living,
Desiring to quit, give up, throw in the towel.
Insecure, I would often vacillate,
Unsure of any path that I might take.
I felt unspoken judgment from others looking on.
If they could only feel the sorrow of my silent song.

## SOMETIMES

Sometimes there's a day when my hope sparks bright,
Then my heart is glad, I can see the light.
Then ambition soars to its highest peak,
And my mind's great store is from sleep released.
Sometimes suddenly, all my hopes fall flat.
Then my heart is sad; confidence I lack.
Then ambition's doors are all closed shut,
And my mind's great store is not worth so much.

## MY PILLOW AND ME

When darkness falls and silence reigns,
When shadows creep on window panes,
When men and infants go to rest
And day birds all are in their nests,
To me come thoughts of grief and woe
And no one but my pillow knows.

When children dream their happy dreams
Of candy bars and chocolate creams,
When lovers sleep in tranquil ease
And all around is blessed peace,
Alone, I lay awake and think,
Of madness I am on the brink.

When thoughts delirious fill my mind
And heartaches make me wince and pine,
When tears fall hot upon my cheek
And sobbing leaves me faint and weak,
My pillow, although wet with tears,
Is still immune to all my fears.

When tremors shake my body taut
And I from weeping am distraught,
When maddening pain shoots through my head
And I lay wishing I were dead,
No words of comfort, none of cheer,
For no one knows and no one cares.

Then when at last fatigued and worn
I lay in troubled sleep at morn,
From ugly dream I soon awake
And once again with sobs I shake.
And through it all, who's there to see?
No one but my pillow and me! 1972

"The Lord upholds all those who fall and lifts up all who are bowed down...the Lord is near to all who call on him, to all who call on him in truth...he hears their cry and saves them."
Psalm 145:14, 18, 19

## JAMAICA I MUST BID FAREWELL

Jamaica I must bid farewell
Though with a heavy heart,
Few years ago I could not tell
That we would have to part;
But oh how oft' in this short life
When we would have our way
Circumstance maps out a path
And we must in it stay.

We all are slaves to Circumstance
But on the other hand
He is no less a slave for he
Must do as God commands.
I would and yet I would not stay,

The urge both ways is strong;
But I'm afraid that if I stay
I would be doing wrong.

For if God has a plan for me,
That plan I cannot spurn.
And if I do not go, I may
My back on blessings turn.
And yet I love my island home.
I would not leave its shore,
But wish that God had willed me
Here to stay forevermore. 1972

"Have I not commanded you? Be strong and courageous. Do not be terrified; do not be dismayed, for the Lord your God will be with you wherever you go." Joshua 1:9

# PART 2. CHANGING VISTAS

## *SELF-PITY ISLAND*

Alone on Self-Pity Island
I sat in my misery,
Waiting for someone to stop by
Who would sit and cry with me.
As I wept I murmured
Against God and His dealings with me.
I was losing my physical vision
And my spiritual acuity.

The soil on Self-Pity Island
Made fertile by my tears
Gave birth to discontentment
Which so many people ensnares.
As I wept it flourished
And overshadowed me
And soon Self-Pity Island
Was covered with this dread tree.

Such gloom my life pervaded
As soul and sight grew dim.
"Death must be better than this," I mused,
I was grieving deep within.
Then as though someone stood near me,
A voice came soft, yet clear,
"Weep not, just count your blessings
And cast on God your cares!"

Startled, I looked around me
But saw no one there.
I stood for a moment in silence
As the words rang in my ears.

I surely had forgotten
All the blessings that were mine
And the more I thought about them,
The more I seemed to find.

Discovering many talents
That had laid latently,
I knew God had a reason,
That He had a plan for me.
I saw how I could comfort
Or encourage some lonely heart,
So I left Self-Pity Island
Bound for a brand new start.

On my journey I've met people
Who have lost all their sight,
And I've been so strongly reminded
That to murmur I have no right.
Occasionally it seems my fears
And woes would weigh me down;
I sometimes sit around and cry
Or else will wear a frown.

My brooding is often disrupted
By another's plea for help,
And I find that in giving comfort
I am comforted myself.
So if this is my role in life, Lord,
I pray that Your will be done.
May I, like my name, bring joy and cheer
To the people I walk among. 1973

"I will lead the blind by ways they have not known, along
unfamiliar paths I will guide them; I will turn the darkness into light
before them and make the rough places smooth. These are the things
I will do; I will not forsake them." Isaiah 42:16

# IN SEARCH OF JOY

After returning to the United States as a legal resident in 1973, I attended Saint Paul's Rehabilitation Center for the Blind. Group 63 was a class of individuals receiving training in mobility, techniques of daily living, and psychosocial adjustment to complete or partial loss of sight. We were a motley crew with few things in common besides vision loss. Humor often rescued us from the pit of depression. Before we separated, I wrote a hilarious poem highlighting the idiosyncrasies of each group member. I have fond memories of a schoolteacher from Kenya, who recoiled in horror when first offered a hot dog. We roared with laughter while explaining that it wasn't actually a dog.

The idea of using a cane was repulsive at first. Everybody would know I was *different;* I wouldn't be able to hide. As I learned mobility with the white cane, I began to appreciate how much independence would be achieved. I stuffed my fears, though they surfaced intermittently. Eric Sollee, the shop instructor and fencing coach, introduced us to the art of fencing. In the woodworking shop, I learned to use power tools safely, then designed and built a bookcase for my 18-volume Braille Bible. The lower section had sliding doors, concealing smaller shelves for my cassettes and related paraphernalia.

As the only participant who already knew Braille, I blossomed in self-confidence. When the program ended, I applied to college and enrolled in several courses with Hadley Correspondence School for the Blind to improve my Braille skills. My first formal use of Braille occurred when I took the Stanford Achievement Test the following year.

Eight years after high school, I was granted a full scholarship to Springdale College. I received a Perkins Brailler and a reel-to-reel tape recorder, my trusted tools for the next four years, along with a Smith Corona typewriter, a hand magnifier, and a cassette player. Before the influx of low-vision technology and talking computers, Braille was my dependable companion. The reel-to-reel tape recorder has been obsolete for many years, but that Perkins Brailler is still working.

Recordings for the Blind provided textbooks, while paid student and volunteer readers assisted with research. Tests were sometimes oral, as I was quizzed by the professor or a grad student. It was impossible to complete all examinations under the same time constraints as sighted students, so I often had take-home exams. Demanding though it was, I made the Dean's list every year and received the *Student-of-the-Year* award from Recordings for the Blind in my junior year. I was also nominated to *Who's Who Among Students.* At age 30, I graduated Magna Cum Laude with a BA degree in Rehabilitation Counseling.

"I can do everything through him who gives me strength."
Philippians 4:13

## A GIFT DISCOVERED

As a young girl, I was very shy and insecure, hating to be in the limelight. Just boarding a bus filled with staring eyes caused great anxiety. During elocution class in high school, I was always petrified when it was my turn to speak. After my first speech class in college, I whined to the professor, "I can't do this," but he didn't let me off the hook. Agonizing through the ordeal, I ended the course with an "A" and somewhat improved self-confidence. The sociology professor refused to give me an "A" for my first course. Can you guess why? I hadn't participated in class discussion. With great effort, I made the grade the following trimester.

Several students from the college attended a local church in Springdale, along with staff from Campus Ministry, who were our spiritual mentors. When asked to share my Christian testimony, I was somewhat apprehensive. Nevertheless, understanding that my life's primary purpose was to honor God, I accepted the invitation. After laboring over my speech with much anxiety, I mounted the platform, heart pounding and hands shaking. Shaky hands are not conducive to reading Braille. As I spoke, my hands grew steady, and my heart's rhythm slowed. One thing in my favor was that I couldn't see the faces of my audience.

Mama used to say that being born in a Christian home doesn't make you a Christian any more than being born in a garage makes you a car. God doesn't have grandchildren, but commands each person to repent and come to a knowledge of the truth (John 17:17; Acts 4:12). According to Scripture, we are all sinners, condemned and alienated from God (Romans 1:18; 3:23). Because of His great love and mercy, God sent His Son, Jesus, to die for sinners, making reconciliation possible. He raised Jesus from the dead to bring us new life (Romans 5:8; 6:23; 1 Peter 3:18).

Jesus said: "I tell you the truth, whoever hears my word and believes him who sent me has eternal life and will not be condemned; he has crossed over from death to life." (John 5:24; 3:16-18) At age 12, I believed, and in believing, I received new life and the right to become a child of God (John 1:12; 2 Corinthians 5:17, 18). That year, Grace and I were baptized as a public declaration of our faith in Jesus.

Facing the threat of blindness as a teenager, I wrestled with depression and lack of self-confidence. Joy crumbled, and hope grew faint. Drowning in self-pity, I doubted God's love and His promise of an abundant life (John 10:10).

Despite my doubts, God had a plan and began opening my eyes to the gifts He had already given me, showing me how I could find purpose by blessing others. I soon reached the place where I could say, "Lord, I trust Your wisdom and Your love. Work out Your plan, whatever it may be." I clung in faith to God's promise never to forsake me (Hebrews 13:5b). I believed that His plans would secure my future and restore my hope (Jeremiah 29:11). I did not imagine college as a part of His plan, but His ways are not my ways (Isaiah 55:8, 9).

Several people thanked me for sharing. What I remember most was a comment from one of my mentors, "You should speak more, you have a gift." The next time I spoke was at a Christmas conference before an audience of hundreds. Later, I was invited to be the guest speaker and musician at a Christian women's luncheon in Springdale.

Life has been challenging, but my experience of God's faithfulness gives me something meaningful to talk about. He has also provided many opportunities to share the gifts of poetry and music. Even if I sweat a little in anticipation, blessing others blesses me.

"Oh, the depths of the riches of the wisdom and knowledge of God! How unsearchable are his judgements and his paths beyond tracing out! And who has known the mind of the Lord? Or who has been his counselor... For from him and through him and to him are all things." Romans 11:33, 34, 36

## A GRADUATE'S TRIBUTE TO HER BEST FRIEND

I have been successful, won many victories,
Accomplished, attained and new heights gained.
Some people call it courage or inner motivation.
They give me all the credit, yet I cannot take it.
They mean well, Lord, but just don't understand
The pact that You and I have made,
So all the praise and glory I pass along to You.
Lord, I know I have come this far only by trusting You,
And without You I can go no further.
You have answered my soul's deepest cries
In moments when I couldn't even verbalize my fears.
In times of need, I've thrown myself on You,
And You have never turned me away.
You have seen my tears and gently wiped them away;
You have known my insecurities, my strivings to become,
And in Your love, You've embraced me,
A frightened, floundering, misguided girl,
Forgiven and made me Your very own.

You have blessed my life in ways that are unspeakable,
In ways that only You and I will ever know!
You are indeed my dearest friend!
Knowing what others did not know, still You loved me.
You have cared when others could not care;
You have given what others could not give:
Courage and desire to live.
You are to me what no man can ever be,
My inner motivation, my very life!
I gave You my weakness; You replaced it with strength.
I came to you struggling;
You sent me back to face the world, a conqueror!
All that I am and have, You gave.
All that I accomplished, You did!
With a full heart, I thank You for them all!
The battle is not over, for life goes on.
So I must go on to greater exploits.
Lord, I will not take one step without You.
Show me the way and I will walk in it,
For I have proved that Your way leads to victory.
Let my life count for You, and I know that I will live,
Really live, until I die! 1978

## JOY IN MOTION

During my senior year, I thought long and hard about my direction after graduation. Through a series of unexpected events, I decided that my place for the next three years was on staff with a Christian campus ministry. I accepted a job with this organization as a counselor in the Career & Personal Counseling Center of Boylston College. The college years are challenging, and my experience was greatly enhanced through the influence of dedicated Christian mentors. It would be a privilege to help students in similar ways. Staff members received part of our salary from the church or college with which we worked, and raised the rest through donations from family and friends.

On June 18th, I joined 40 new staff members for training. It was difficult making the transition from Springdale, where the faculty had habituated to my needs as a visually impaired person, to an organization unfamiliar with my particular disability. Despite the frustration and tears, God again demonstrated that His grace is sufficient. I met Muriel at a prospective staff meeting in February. She became a great source of encouragement that summer, helping me with reading and shopping. Do you ever have worries or anxieties you don't dare utter for fear of seeming foolish? Can you relate? Well, Muriel could, and every time I dared to share she understood.

Staff training included Evangelism and Discipleship. Some students made their first commitment to the Lord Jesus; others were renewed in their faith. It was exciting to hear these students share their testimonies. I attended seminars on Biblical Counseling, the Christian World View, and Inductive Bible Study. Orientation to the Counseling Center at Boylston began in July. I worked with two groups of high school students in a Life/Career Planning Seminar, then rejoined the other staff. A week later, we moved camp to a Bible conference center in Morris Town. The schedule was lighter, and I stayed with a family, enjoying home-cooked meals, a welcome change! The lectures were on the person and work of Christ, with rap sessions on the relevance of Christianity to everyday life.

Old and new staff united for the grand finale week, a highlight of which was the banquet held for interested parents and friends. I was encourage by the response to my poem, "Self-Pity Island." A gesture of love made by the staff touched me deeply. I owned a Braille Bible, but needed a concordance to help with in-depth study. It was casually mentioned to a few individuals, one of whom brought it to the attention of the other staff members. As a result, I received the gift of a 10-volume Braille concordance.

When training ended, my new roommate and I made the big move to Boylston. Liz had been on staff for one year and worked in the counseling center. We had one week to get settled and report to work. It was hectic, as we unpacked, cleaned, and ran to furniture stores and yard sales in search of bargains. Our spacious three-bedroom, split-level rental was only $150 a month. We each had a study, and there was a fireplace, for which Liz had specifically prayed. The house came unfurnished, but we received furniture from unexpected sources. God was so good to us! We dedicated the house to His service. It was about a 15-minute walk from the school, far enough for students or staff who needed a retreat from the noisy campus.

As the new school year began, I was again on the college scene, not as a student, but as an anxious staff member. Of course, my status as a student of life had not changed, for every day is a new adventure. Boylston was new territory, but the friendly atmosphere reminded me of Springdale. I was warned about the winters, so with all the new beginnings, my old dread of the cold remained.

April, 1979

Dear Friends,

While hibernating in below zero weather, being in love, and weathering some unexpected changes, I continue to impact the lives of students. Brighton House, an arm of the counseling center, caters to at-risk freshman, providing extra help in basic study skills and habits. We also provide personal and group counseling, tutoring, and testing.

Chip became a Christian shortly before Christmas and has been meeting with me regularly for Bible study and personal counseling. Most people who knew him in the fall will readily admit that his life has changed dramatically. He quit smoking; his language is cleaner; his self-confidence has increased, and he desires to practice his new faith in sincerity. I have been building relationships with several members of Beulah Baptist Church. In February the pastor invited me to speak and play my accordion on a television broadcast. Jealous of my celebrity, my brother wondered if the station went out of business after showing my face.

During the past few months, I have been grappling with the unexpected turn of events regarding my job. Already discouraged by the lack of certain necessary accommodations, I also learned that, funds will not be available to pay my salary after August. This was disconcerting until I regained perspective. God is still in control. He has carried me through many trials and will only use this to grow my trust in Him.

A few years ago, while working on an inner-city project, I became interested in a young man. We have maintained a long-distance relationship, and he recently visited me in Boylston. We have agreed that the friendship holds promise, and wish to take the next step.

I am considering a Master's in counseling at Radcliffe Seminary. Through a partnership with this campus ministry, I have already earned some credits from our staff training. If my plans solidify, I will be moving to California. My beau just happens to live there. I need your continued financial support for ongoing ministry expenses and the cost of moving at the end of the school year. Your prayers and letters of encouragement will be greatly appreciated during this transition.

I eagerly anticipate the next adventure God has planned for me.

"In their hearts humans plan their course, but the Lord establishes their steps." Proverbs 16:9

Joy

## *I LOVE THE MAN*

I love the man, my heart so yearns
Just to be with him where he is.
I love the man and yet must wait
For the divine sanction of Thy will.
I love the man and feel You've given
Your confirmation deep within,
And yet, like Abraham Your friend,
I hope and doubt and hope again.
Yet to him, your promise was fulfilled,
So like him, I am trusting still.
I love the man and so must wait
With patience till the time is full.
You've planted this desire in me,
And so I pray, Lord, let it be!
I do believe, so strengthen me
And clear away the unbelief;
Grant the desire of my heart,
Bring him to me, Lord, at last. 1979

# PART 3. DREAMS REDEFINED

## CALIFORNIA, HERE I COME

August 2, 1979

Dear Friends,

Greetings from sunny California! The move from Boylston became a reality sooner than expected. I thank the Lord for my boss, who generously granted me two months' vacation with pay. This greatly facilitated the move to Los Angeles.

The cost of living here is high, so finding employment is crucial. I have contacted a vocational counselor from the Rehab Department to assist with job placement. For the last month, I have been sharing an apartment with two Christian sisters, but I will eventually have to find my own place. Please pray for God to open the right doors.

Thank you for your faithful support, which helped me through a tough year. I am sure that God has used me in more ways than are evident right now. The good times and friendships, as well as the growing pains, have enhanced my faith. I know that I can indeed trust Him with my life, present and future. In January I panicked, uncertain of where I would be going or how I would get there. Here I am, six months later, with high aspirations for the future. I hope that my life, with all its ups and downs, can be an example of God's faithfulness and love. If you are facing hardship, be encouraged. Remember, His faithfulness and love remain constant even when we are faithless. It is our unbelief that affects our ability to receive what He has to give.

"...shout for joy. For the word of the Lord is right and true; he is faithful in all he does...the earth is full of his unfailing love."
Psalm 33:3-5

## SONG OF JOY

When you were born, the angels sang.
I was too young to recognize the hour's significance,
So the angels sang for Joy!
The song grew in beauty as you grew in stature,
Reaching resounding crescendo when you were born anew!
For there is great rejoicing over every soul that finds the Lord.

Years passed in silence, dreams hazy and vague
Void of any background music.
Unknowingly, we were wending our ways toward each other
And soon the silence was broken.
Strains of a lilting melody filled my ears and stirred my heart.
A peculiar excitement gripped me!
The music seemed to come from Heaven, yet was within,
Responding to my soul's sad soliloquies.
This was the melody my dreams had lacked
Now emerging into glorious sound.
My heart in confidence picked up the strain
And then, o happy day!
I saw you and knew!

My heart sang a refrain till then inaudible:
"This, this is he for whom your heart has longed.
Behold the man who shall complete your joy!
Yes, this is the man to whom your heart belongs!"
And from that day, my Sweetheart,
The song the angels sang became my own.
The sad soliloquies ceased as your soul dialogued with mine,
Enhancing the melody with new dimensions,
Creating beauty that makes angels listen in hushed amazement
As we shake Heaven with the melody of our nuptial song!

# JOYFUL ANNOUNCEMENT

January 24, 1980

Dear Friends,

Although I had applied for rehab services in July, mobility orientation did not begin until October. I am still unemployed, but learning to get around town on my own has done wonders for my self-confidence. A few weeks before Christmas, I finally moved into my own apartment. Having my own space, with boxes unpacked, has restored a sense of being in control. While waiting, I found an outlet for my frustration by refinishing used furniture now sitting attractively in my apartment. From that experience I have coined a new proverb: "Necessity nurtures creativity."

Now for a real surprise! Three and a half years ago, I met my prince, a tall (6'4"), dark and handsome man. Prince Charming, a native of California, home of the stars, was unaware that he was destined to tie the Gordian knot that would make him mine forever. Our friendship, nurtured across thousands of miles, has blossomed into a love relationship. We proudly announce our engagement! Since I am a foot shorter than my Prince, I take the liberty to suggest a stepladder or sturdy footstool as the ideal wedding gift. Such a gift could save on medical expenses that I may incur from neck and back strain in my attempts to embrace the Prince.

On a more serious note, we have already encountered some of the conflicts natural to this kind of relationship. Aware of the significance and solemnity of the step we are about to take, we need your prayers. Pray that God will give us the courage, wisdom and determination to keep our commitment firm.

Floating on air,

Joy

# NEW BLESSINGS

August, 1980

Dear Friends,

We did it! The knot has been tied! In March we had a brief ceremony at a local church. It was attended by close friends and my hubby's immediate family. Edward, a former spiritual mentor, stood in as proxy for my father, and Wanda, a college friend, was my maid of honor.

My large family couldn't afford traveling expenses to attend our wedding in California, so in July, my parents graciously hosted a formal reception for us in Boston. It was like having a second wedding. I'm probably one of the few brides who got to wear her bridal gown twice. My sisters, Grace, Carol and Faith, were bridesmaids, and my friend, Muriel, the maid of honor. My brothers, Paul, Danny, and two family friends, escorted the ladies. While still in the area, my hubby and I also managed to squeeze in a visit to Springdale, my old stomping grounds.

A week before the wedding, I began working as a Braille and communication skills instructor. Optimum Living Center (OLC) is a residential center for blind and developmentally disabled adults. The Department of Rehabilitation supplied me with various low-vision devices that increased my competence on the job. I could have used these services at Boylston. The most revolutionary of these is a Closed-Circuit Television (CCTV), an electronic visual aid system featuring a 19-inch monitor equipped with a camera that magnifies print. This enhances my ability to teach reading to the partially-sighted students. Managing paperwork, both job-related and personal, is much easier. I am also able to write legibly on lined paper, read my handwriting, sign checks and even view photos. Imagine my excitement!

The process is tedious, but my dependence on others has decreased considerably, though not completely. It is gratifying to read a personal letter at my own convenience and in privacy (as long as the letter is typed or the handwriting is legible). My heart is overflowing with gratitude for the increased autonomy and self-assurance that this technological creation provides.

"I will praise the Lord all my life; I will sing praise to my God as long as I live." Psalm 146:2

## PROTECT THIS MAN

Protect this man from deeds of darkness,
May he daily practice acts of kindness,
Encircle him with Your angels of light,
Direct his steps as he walks in the night.

In a mixed-up, hurting world, oh Lord,
Grant peace and comfort from Your Word,
When he falters at choosing right, oh God,
Uphold him with Your power from above.

When he feels life isn't worth the fight,
Lord, You set his perspective right;
Increase wisdom, fortitude and faith
As Your awesome love he contemplates.

Give purpose to him each step of the way,
Keep his passions under your powerful sway,
Protect him from hate and greed and lust,
With his whole heart, may he in You trust.

Firm commitment, love, and integrity
May all men in his dealings see.
May he persevere though the race is long,
May he find joy as he conquers wrong. 1980

This is dedicated to the man I love!

# ADJUSTING TO LIFE

January 5, 1982

Dear Friends,

A happy and prosperous New Year to you all! I decided not to send Christmas cards since a newsletter after the hustle and bustle would serve my purposes better. We had nine guests for Christmas dinner, including a family of four from El Salvador and a student from OLC. My Spanish got some needed practice. Hubby and I spent the New Year weekend enjoying each other and discussing our goals for 1982.

Speaking of goals, last year I decided to work on at least one creative project each month. Between macramé plant hangers, latch hook rugs, stuffed toys, handmade Christmas ornaments and pillows, I far exceeded the quota. I am thankful the Creator of the universe has chosen to share His creativity with me. One of the highlights of the year was my new sewing machine. I still haven't figured out how to thread the needle without help, but I am planning to take sewing classes at the Braille Institute.

Some of you have requested more information about my Prince. He was involved in campus ministry as a student leader, and we met while working in an inner-city ministry with other college students. He is a man of few words, but loves the written word. He was an English major, so our apartment is always overrun with books, newspapers, magazines and pamphlets. He was out of work for most of last year, but is now temporarily employed as an inspector of Mediterranean fruit flies. That infestation wasn't all bad, after all; one man's pest proved to be another man's provision. He is also a very good cook, and calls me his fiery Jamaican woman when I get angry.

Last year, I struggled with anger and resentment regarding problems at work. My supervisor's behavior was spreading discord and alienating people. It wasn't easy, but I approached her with an attitude of love. She thanked me for caring enough to confront her.

This was a major victory because I am not usually that bold. Bitterness left my heart, and unnecessary tension was released, allowing me to better cope with normal work pressures.

Our pastor, in a series of messages on the family, emphasized the need for a Christian marriage to be Christ-centered. Only Jesus can unite two individuals who are basically sinful and selfish. Each partner has a God-given responsibility, which must be carried out as unto the Lord. Each must seek to become a better mate rather than trying to make one's mate better. If I trust God's promise to meet my needs, then I can be free to seek my mate's welfare instead of being overly preoccupied with mine. We want to live out these principles and know we can do it only with God's strength.

"Do nothing out of selfish ambition or vain conceit. Rather, in humility, value others above yourselves, not looking to your own interests but each of you to the interests of the others."
Philippians 2:3, 4

# ANTICIPATED JOY

November 10, 1982

Dear Friends,

I cannot share the sentiments of women who say pregnancy was the best time of their life. Mine has been miserable with incessant morning sickness, yet the doctor's report is always positive. We seem to struggle hardest for the things that are dearest. Nevertheless, as the Lord Jesus endured the cross in joyful anticipation of bringing new life to us, so He has enabled me to endure my pregnancy and now we joyfully await the birth of our baby.

This year, we have been poignantly reminded that our trust should not be in the economy or our bank account, but in God whose resources never run dry. We are both presently unemployed, but God has faithfully provided. In addition to job hunting, my hubby has been investing more time in Bible study. He has been very loving and supportive at a time when I really need it.

Last May, Grace, her husband and son came from Jamaica along with my maternal grandmother. This was Aunt Adah's first trip to the states since our family migrated. We celebrated Patrick's marriage, my nephew's third birthday, Carol's graduation from college, and my pregnancy. Daniel lives in the Northwest. Paul is still at home. Faith, the baby, is a junior in college.

As the awesome responsibility of parenting begins, we need your prayers more than ever. In a world where the distinction between right and wrong is rapidly disappearing, and where there is increasing distortion of moral issues, we are greatly in need of God's wisdom. We desire to be the kind of parents that will uphold His standards. Please pray for us and have a blessed Christmas!

## TIDINGS OF GREAT JOY

Hi, my name is Avizi. I was born in December at 1:04 AM. I weighed seven pounds, six ounces and was 21 inches long. Mommy had to have an emergency C-section, but we are both fine now. Grandma Walker came from Boston to help Mommy and Daddy. I took my time coming, so she had to wait three whole weeks before I was born.

Everybody says I'm a handsome boy and look just like Daddy. It must be true because all the ladies go crazy when they see me. Mommy is very busy between feeding me and changing my diapers and doesn't get enough sleep. I know she loves every moment of it and wouldn't trade me for anything in the whole world. She says I am a treasure from God. That means I'm very special.

"For you created my inmost being; you knit me together in my mother's womb. I praise you because I am fearfully and wonderfully made; your works are wonderful, I know that full well. My frame was not hidden from you when I was made in the secret place…Your eyes saw my unformed body; all the days ordained for me were written in your book before one of them came to be." Psalm 139:13-16

# MOM'S MEMORIES

Dear Son,

I loved you before I knew you, while you were still growing in my womb. I prayed for God to guard your life, to make you wise, to bring me joy through you. I wanted you to be strong and independent. I felt you kick so many times and knew you would be strong. You were practicing your football kicks even in my womb.

Preparing to be the best mom, I read the baby books as I anticipated your entrance into my world. I made your crib sheets and bumper pads from colorful fabric to stimulate you, and adorned your crib with stuffed animals made with my own hands. I was so excited about your coming!

When labor began, the pain was intense. I was just a few centimeters dilated when your heart rate began to decrease. The doctors were concerned, and I was really scared.

Thank God! They cut me open to save you. I lost two babies before you and one after you. Clearly, God intended you to be born. In medicated stupor, I barely saw you before they whisked you away to the neonatal unit, where you spent the next five days. You had your first bowel movement in utero and had aspirated the meconium.

The next morning, your dad wheeled me to the NCU. As I held you, gazing with wonder while whispering your name, big brown eyes looked back at me with obvious recognition. The tenderness I felt was indescribable. My son! My boy! My joy! Your Daddy, Grandma and the nurses were all admiring you, when their voices seemed to slowly fade away. My mommy radar kicked in. I cried "take the baby" and passed out.

I kept you safe for nine long months and couldn't let you fall. My job was to protect you; I didn't want you hurt at all. There was a great hubbub about me having a seizure. I think I was just tired and hungry after labor and surgery. The doctors ordered all kinds of tests to be sure I wouldn't take them to the bank. This kept me from having to go home without you. Five days later, your Daddy brought us home. You were healthy, and we were very happy.

I held you close and nursed you, experiencing a new mom's euphoria. You had been introduced to a bottle in the neonatal unit, but I persisted in breast-feeding you even through those painful bites. I never imagined that toothless gums could grip so tight. I sometimes pumped the milk into a bottle to provide me some relief. Knowing that breast-feeding was the best way to grow a healthy baby, I persevered for 11 months. I wanted what was best for you, whatever it might cost me. You were my joy, and I was your mom.

You were a gift from God, so we would cherish and raise you to love Him. I have prayed continually to that end. I prayed for wisdom to mold you into the image of God and for strength to be a good example. I prayed for protection from harmful influences, for soundness of mind, body and spirit.

When you were only two, God inspired me to homeschool you. With my visual impairment, I didn't know how I would accomplish it, but God, who qualifies the called, gave me the wherewithal. I poured my life into you, championing your cause. I bathed you, fed you, played with you, and sang to you. I rocked you when you were howling and watched while you were sleeping.

Just days after a third miscarriage, I almost lost you. Your eyes rolled back in your head as you stiffened in my arms. I screamed to God, "Please don't take my baby!" He heard my cry and saved you. What would I have done without you, my pride, my joy, my son, my boy?

Your sister was born when you were three years old. You immediately became her protective big brother. When the nurse pricked her heel to check for keturnuria, you told her, very firmly, "Don't hurt my sister." You would stare at her through the crib bars, waiting expectantly for her to "wake up and play." You loved her so much. One day, when her diaper leaked, to my astonishment, you offered to clean it up. You were so helpful!

Of course there were the moments of sibling rivalry. When your sister was about six months old and sitting up, I placed her on the floor with you. A few minutes later, she was screaming. When I asked what had happened, your answer was a dead giveaway: "She fell down and hit her head three times." The day you cut a chunk out of her hair, I thought her hair was falling out until we found the scissors. Your dad taped the hair and scissors to the door and waited until you were awake next morning. When we pointed to it, you just hung your head.

Your daddy often scolded me for letting pins fall on the floor while I was sewing. "What if Avizi puts them in his mouth?" Well, the first time you found a pin, you found my butt and stuck it in. I yelped; you laughed! You were a smart little brat!

I carried you on my back for a long time, even after you learned to walk. It was much simpler than trying to push a stroller while using my white cane. As you got older, we often walked around the neighborhood while you chattered away. We were so close then. How the years have changed things. Now I carry you in my heart.

"Sons are a heritage from the Lord, children a reward from him."
Psalm 127:3

## A MAN AFTER GOD'S OWN HEART

My child, treasure wisdom, not this world's kind,
But the wisdom that issues from God's mind.
Let God be your personal Friend and Guide
And through all of life He'll be at your side.

His wisdom will help you make the right choices,
Know what to shun and heed the right voices.
So we pray that in your youthful days,
You will seek God first and walk in His ways.

He will help you fight against sin,
Struggle through difficult times and win;
And when you lose, He'll still be there
Granting you grace and compassionate care.

He'll show you how to be a good friend,
How to love others and a helping hand lend.
He'll make you strong, yet gentle and kind,
For such is the wisdom that comes from God's mind.

Seek first God's kingdom, not fortune or fame,
Pursue pure wisdom, not ill-gotten gain;
Learn to love Jesus right from the start,
And He'll make you a man after God's own heart.

"The wisdom that comes from heaven is first of all pure; then peace-loving, considerate, submissive, full of mercy and good fruit, impartial and sincere." James 3:17

## YOU ARE BLACK

My son, you are Black and you'd better be proud!
Don't hang your Black head or get lost in the crowd.
Don't buy the white lie some men like to spin;
They say you are "less than," but that is a sin!
For God made you special when He selected your shade,
And my son, since God made you, then you are well made!
So don't let nobody tell you wrong!
It's okay to be Black, my son!

Your Black ancestors fought hard and long
Because they knew slavery was wrong.
They fought for freedom and dignity,
And you must still fight perpetually;
For even though slavery is no more,
Racism is still outside your door.

But don't let nobody tell you wrong!
It's okay to be Black, my son!

Now don't be afraid to go outside,
'Cause your Blackness is nothing you need to hide.
Display the gifts with which you're endowed,
Of your Black heritage, always be proud!
Show your Black face, hold your Black head high,
Maintain your dignity or die!
And don't let nobody tell you wrong!
It's mighty fine to be Black, my son! 1983

## MY CALLING

When my son was a toddler, I heard a leading advocate of homeschooling discussing his basic philosophy. He highlighted the superiority of one-to-one instruction, and that parents are best equipped to teach their values to their offspring. Home teaching can focus on the child's individual learning style and affords more time for promoting creativity and non-academic learning. He further indicated that too many parents abdicate their God-given responsibilities, believing the myth that someone else is more equipped to prepare their children for life. The common sense of the idea grabbed me. I knew then that my calling was to homeschool my son.

Shortly after my daughter was born, I convinced my husband to attend a workshop with me. The speaker felt that children are, by nature, antisocial and cannot socialize each other. In a room full of six-year-olds, all we have is what he called "pooled ignorance." It is the proper interaction with an adult that teaches a child social skills. When children spend most of their waking hours with someone else, it is more difficult for parents to transmit their values to them. My husband thought homeschooling was radical, and I supposed it was, yet I was more persuaded than ever.

In searching for materials suitable for a visually impaired mother, I discovered Play & Talk, a phonics program which included both audio and printed materials. Knowing that reading would be the foundation of all learning (and with something to prove), I started teaching Avizi to read. Meanwhile, I had met other homeschool families in my area and joined a support group. One of the moms gave me a beginning reader to test my son, who was then five years old. His dad and I were excited at his motivation. Our son was reading! I had proven my point and would continue what I had begun.

Contrary to my own private apprehensions, my visual impairment did not hamper my children in any way. Eager to help and eager to learn, both became avid readers, a direct result of having to assist Mom. They would spell the labels on spices and other items. As their competence grew, so did their pride in reading the lists of ingredients on boxes and bottles. From this came an early interest in cooking, as they learned to bake and prepare simple meals.

When Avizi started reading, I gave him books with arts & crafts projects. He read and delivered. What a fulfilling way for a mother to spend her day! I didn't have to wait for the babysitter or teacher to tell me what my child had discovered. I was there when it happened. I helped make it happen. There were even times when it happened without me, but I was there to share in the joy of discovery.

There were many critics at first. A relative repeatedly asked me when I would start sending the children to school. I replied, "They are in school!" She didn't get it then, but I have lived to hear her congratulate me on a job well done. A schoolteacher friend once patronizingly suggested that she understood I wanted to keep the children at home because I was lonely. What a joke! Not long after, she hailed me.

"Joy, wait, I need to talk to you. What materials are you using with Avizi? He was reading in Sunday school today. He is an excellent reader! You are doing a great job!"

Most critics of homeschooling have a common concern — socialization. They think that homeschool means sitting at home staring at the walls and never interacting with others. No way! We participated in a support group with scheduled park days, inspiring field trips, and group activities. In our first group, families took turns selecting and setting up various art and science projects for a cooperative learning center held once a month.

Moms moved between stations, reading the instructions and helping their children to complete the projects. I remember one mother's amazement when she saw my son reading the instructions to me instead of me reading to him. Avizi was six years old. Our family's learning center project was about disabilities. I displayed my CCTV, Braillewriter, talking watch, and other low-vision devices. The students were eager to have their names written in Braille and walk with my cane while blindfolded.

After receiving an inquiry from our local school district, my husband and I joined the Homeschool Legal Defense Fund, an organization that protects the rights of homeschooling families. We also enrolled in the Home Education Department of a Christian school. Our children took SAT exams and met with other homeschoolers for Picture Day, Park Day, Graduation Day and other group events. Parents were required to submit lesson plans for accountability. There was never a dull moment.

One year, along with a small group of Black homeschool families, we attended a series of science classes taught by an African-American scientist. Another mom, who had a biology degree, converted her garage into a classroom and held classes for several families. For one of the science projects, each child had the outline of his body drawn on butcher paper. As we studied different organs of the body, the students would color and cut out a picture of that organ, then glue it in its proper place on the butcher paper outline. I loved that practical hands-on approach.

Teaching math was more challenging for me. Besides Standard English Braille, there is also a Braille system for math and science called the Nemeth Code. During the summer, I spent many hours with a friend, transcribing the math curriculum into Braille. Because I hadn't learned the Nemeth Code, I created my own Braille symbols. It was challenging but worked well.

Homeschooling was not easy; however, I would not have traded those years for anything. Every commitment has its less glorious moments, yet I cannot imagine a more fulfilling job.

# JOY IN THE LIBRARY

In elementary school, the bookmobile came once a month. I looked forward to browsing the new selections. When I was older, I frequented the Tom Redcam (Macdermot spelled backwards) Library, named after the first poet laureate of Jamaica. Little did I know the day would come when my ability to peruse the written word would be eclipsed. Fairy tales, as well as Greek and Roman mythology, were high on my list of favorites. I loved the Nancy Drew, Hardy Boys and Judy Bolton mysteries and "Poems for Pleasure."

During high school, I spent most Saturdays at the library. Friday nights were devoted to chores so I could be free on Saturday. With six siblings, it was much easier to do homework and study for exams away from home.

Without modern amenities, chores were not as simple as they are today. I alternated with Grace, scrubbing the floors on our hands and knees with a coconut brush. Other chores included hand-washing clothes, making starch from scratch, starching, and pressing school uniforms with irons heated on a coal stove. I was often tired and would doze off before starting the rigors of studying. Sometimes a girlfriend or two would meet me at the library.

Miss Carrington was the high school librarian. She also taught Latin, one of my better subjects. As her assistant, I rescued books from destructive bookworms by painting each one with a protective chemical. This gave me more time with my favorite teacher and was a great way to acquaint myself with the volumes in the library.

As my vision deteriorated, and reading became more challenging, the idea of going to a library produced more frustration than pleasure. After being declared legally blind, I discovered the world of Talking Books. Although I read Braille, I prefer audio books when reading for pleasure. Today it is impossible for me to walk into a public library and even read the titles of audio books. I sometimes feel a quiet impatience with the person helping me. He or she is selectively reading titles aloud. I don't know what is being omitted. In Los Angeles, where I now reside, the Braille Institute Library provides recorded books for the blind and visually impaired. I need only call and request a book. They are sent to me in the mail, or I can pick them up in person. Entering this library does not leave me feeling helpless, but it does take time for new releases to be recorded, so there is still some frustration when I desire to read a current release. However, the Braille Institute also has a volunteer service that will record a book on request, if I provide the printed copy.

When the children were young, my frustration was keen whenever I entered a library. I couldn't select books for them without the librarian's assistance. On discovering an interesting book, my son would spell difficult words as he read to me. Losing library books was frustrating, so developing a home library became a priority. Putting Braille labels on the first few books gave me a sense of being in charge. I stocked our library with books on a wide range of topics and reading levels. My aim was to stimulate their interests and to develop a varied vocabulary.

Soon, we had so many books, making Braille labels was neither time nor cost-effective. I lost my sense of control until my discovery of Braille-Print books produced by National Braille Press. We could then read to each other. The children's growing love of reading brought me much pleasure. My goal had been accomplished. I recall my son asking for new books; he had "read every book in the house twice."

Although entering a public library today still reminds me of my limitations, I recognize that those constraints have taught me to be resourceful. The challenge of homeschooling helped me find ways to circumvent roadblocks. Despite visual impairment, I taught my fully sighted children to love and master reading, a vital skill in a visual world.

# TESTED AND TRIED

February 2, 1985

Dear Friends,

Last year, various personal upheavals made life very stressful and painful. I often had to shut down my emotions just to cope, not a condition conducive to letter writing. Besides, a newsletter is a luxury we can barely afford. Being a mother and homemaker also keeps me very busy.

Another miscarriage left me disappointed and angry with God. Why didn't He protect my baby when so many women are destroying theirs deliberately? I was afraid to admit my anger and went numb instead. Through counseling, I was reminded that I could acknowledge my feelings to God; I didn't need to pretend. I was angry with Him because I didn't grasp how much He understood my pain. I was also reminded that we live in a fallen, sin-cursed world. Christians are not immune to the consequential pain and suffering that is all around us, yet God promises to be with us through it all. We have not given up. As soon as I get my body in shape, we will try again.

Three days after the miscarriage, Avizi developed a very high fever, which led to a seizure. I was terrified! The timing couldn't have been worse. I thought I would lose him too. Thank God he overcame it and hasn't given us a scare like that since. It is fascinating to watch him grow. He turned two in December, has a keen interest in books and loves to sing. When we go to the library, he gets to choose his books, always based on the pictures, of course. He is a loving, happy child, and we are thankful.

Last April, we made a necessary and expeditious move to a larger apartment next door. Since we have the same landlord, we did not have to pay a deposit, but the 85% increase in our rent has put a considerable strain on our budget. In addition, my husband's work hours continue to fluctuate due to budget cuts. He rarely works an eight-hour day and was laid off temporarily last November. His efforts to find other employment have met with failure. We are certainly learning to walk by faith and not by sight (2 Corinthians 5:7).

The stress of unpaid bills and unmet needs is great, but God's loving care is still evident. We sometimes come close to running out of food, yet never do. Some of you have sent us gifts that came right on time even without your awareness of our situation. It gets tough, but we can't give up. Victory may be just around the corner.

Presented with a wardrobe crisis due to excessive weight gain, I joined a sewing class at the local high school and have been making my own clothes. The sewing instructor was challenged to help me find a way to thread the machine independently. How do I manage? Blood, sweat, tears and sheer determination. I have corrugated fingers for all the times I stab myself with a pin or needle or cut myself with the scissors. Nevertheless, it is very rewarding to make something I can wear out the door and receive a compliment.

If sewing is time-consuming for a sighted person, it is doubly so for me. A two-year-old who always wants me to "come play wid de toys" complicates the process. Despite the obstacles, I have replenished my wardrobe and enhanced my self-esteem. I even surprised my hubby with a robe for his birthday. He is always on the lookout for fabric sales, so everything I make is a super bargain. I have made window curtains, as well as an outfit for my toddler.

Thanks to my parents' help, last summer I took Avizi on his first airplane trip to visit my folks. It was an overdue vacation for me. Avizi thoroughly enjoyed his grandparents, aunts and uncles. While we were there, Mama and Daddy left for Jamaica to attend my paternal grandfather's funeral. Pappy was 96.

In spite of the frustrations and demands, I am enjoying motherhood. Avizi is a little chatterbox and can be very amusing. One day he put his jacket over his arm, picked up his book bag and kissed me on the cheek. Heading for the door, he called, "Bye Doy, see you later. Going to wook." He is great for helping me find the pins on the floor when I am sewing. What was not so great was the day he got hold of the scissors and sliced the dress I had just finished making. It hurt, but what could I do?

We wish you a prosperous 1985 in body, soul and spirit, even as we wish it for ourselves. Please keep us in your prayers. Our greatest desire is to trust God and rejoice, no matter how threatening the circumstances. Although I haven't been very good at it this past year, the best way to cope is to remember that "with Christ, in the vessel, we can smile at the storm" (John Newton). We love you!

Joy and family

"Though the fig tree does not bud and there are no grapes on the vine...yet I will rejoice in the Lord, I will be joyful in God my Savior." Habakkuk 3:17, 18

## JOY COMES HOME

March 25, 1986

Dear Friends,

After a miserable pregnancy (I think I hold the world record in vomiting and nausea), I finally went into labor at 4:00 AM, a week after my expected due date. Although I chose a normal delivery, I was considered high risk and prepared for a C-section, just in case. As the contractions grew stronger and longer, I panicked momentarily. Then I felt a surge of strength and calm that could only come from the Lord. I knew that many friends were praying me through. Having my spouse there with his arm on mine was reassuring.

The intensity of the pain was incredible! I considered Eve and what I would like to say to her. At 2:00 PM, I was eight centimeters dilated and no medical problems had arisen. I knew I would make it. At 4:52 PM, a healthy baby girl squirmed her way into the world, squawking her protest. She weighed 8 lbs. 12 oz., was 21 inches long and had a mop of black hair. I was surprisingly alert at her birth, a dramatic contrast to my sedated state when Avizi was delivered. Her daddy commends me for my courage in deciding what I want and then pursuing it with determination. His support is to be highly commended as well.

As we were leaving the hospital, two ladies in the lobby cooed at the baby, calling her a "little angel." Avizi corrected them. "Her not angel, her name Agalia." He has been adjusting very well and is a proud and protective big brother, eager to show off his baby sister to visitors. At her slightest whimper, he comes running, "Mommy, my baby is crying; go pick her up!" Someone remarked that his sister was lucky to have a brother like him. He retorted, frowning, "Her not yucky!" Incidentally, Avizi is now a family man. After I became pregnant, his imaginary friend, Linda, became his wife. They have four kids and a baby. When asked if he goes to school, he replies, "I am a daddy! I go to work. My kids go to school."

Children do bring a lot of pain before, during and after, yet they also bring much joy, and we can't have one without the other. Thanks to all who have supported us with your prayers and gifts. To myself I say, "Be at rest once more, O my soul, for the Lord has been good to you."(Psalm 116:7)

Joy and Family


## AGALIA'S SONG

Do you know that little girl so brown and so pretty?
Do you know that little girl with such big brown eyes?
She has such nice thick braids hanging on her shoulders!
The meaning of her name is: "joy, joy, joy enters the house."
*Agalia!*

Written by Joy & kids

# FLASHBACKS OF JOY

Dear Avizi,

These are flashbacks from a time when we were close, when life was good and laughter flowed freely. They recall eddies of joy and torrents of tears that forged our relationship as mother and son, a relationship that can never be undone.

On our way to church one day, you were talking up a storm in the backseat. We asked, "Who are you talking to?" You responded, "Linda." Curious, we queried, "Who is Linda?" You replied with an air of importance, "She's my wife!" Shortly before Agalia was born, Linda started having babies. You explained that you went under the blanket with Linda. "Her belly got bigger and bigger, and out popped a baby." You were serious; we were stifling the giggles.

You brought so much laughter into my life! I can still picture you sitting in your Daddy's size 15 shoes; you were on your toy telephone, "Linda, send the kids to kool." After your first airplane trip, you were on the phone with Linda again. When we asked where she was, you replied, "She lives over the mountains." I can't recall when Linda faded out of your life, but she eventually did.

My heart was often in my mouth, watching you perform those daredevil stunts on your bicycle. One day you fell and split your lip. You had to get stitches. Oh my goodness! Your screams went through the roof. Each time you got a vaccination, you went wild with panic, and a male nurse had to restrain you.

Born with a slight deformity in your legs, you wore orthopedic shoes for a while. Your tibia was curved inward and your dad wanted the doctor to break and reset your legs. The doctor warned it would be very traumatic, and I agreed. He felt you would outgrow it, and you did. Sometimes you could barely crawl up the stairs because of pain in your legs. You were diagnosed with Osgood Slaughter's disease but outgrew that too.

Nothing stopped you from playing football. Man, you lived and breathed football. I remember you coming home, adrenaline still pumping, enthusiastically rehashing the game for your sister and me. You were all boy.

Your dad and I took you to the Arboretum when you were just a toddler. With colorful tail feathers spread, the peacocks were doing their courtship dance. You were mesmerized. The Arboretum became a frequent haunt during the homeschool years. We sometimes went with Mrs. Gee and her kids. She still remembers, with amusement, when you were excited to see the peacocks and exclaimed, "Mom, look, the apricots!"

Remember those bedtime stories about Francine, who lived in Frankfield with her mom and dad, Frances and Frankenstein, Frank, her brother, and Frankfurter, the dog? The stories were impromptu, and you both loved adding some of the action. One night, as I was telling you a story, I became aware that I was talking gibberish. Apologizing, I explained that I was very tired. You responded tenderly, "It's okay Mommy, I understand."

You enjoyed listening to "Your Story Hour" (all 144 cassettes), absorbing Christian values I wanted you to learn. We were so close then. I miss those days. Remember when you made a dummy with pillows, dressed it in your clothes and left it sitting on my bed? Thinking it was you, I was talking to the dummy, until I heard giggling in the hallway. You and Agalia had a rousing laugh at my expense.

After the Whittier earthquake in 1987, you had trouble sleeping. You would run from your room screaming. I would pray for you and comfort you. Even when you were older, you would ask me to pray with you when you had a bad dream. You knew where to go when there was a problem. I hope you still do.

Mom

## *DO YOUR BEST*

Don't say "I can't" until you have tried,
Until to the task you've some effort applied.
Break the job down into steps that are small,
Then work at each step till you've finished them all.

Pray and ask God for whatever you need,
Ask Him to show you how to succeed.
He can do all and has promised to help,
You can come boldly and ask Him yourself.

Then tackle the job with all that you've got,
Do your best! You can't do better than that.
If after you've tried you still cannot do it,
Just take a break and come back to it.

Don't give up till you've tried again and again,
Don't give up till you're sure you've done all you can.
Then if you find that you really can't do it,
Admit you need help; ask someone for it.

Perhaps there's a person or tool that you need
To make the job easier, to help you succeed.
When you've done all you can, get some help for the rest,
But whatever you do, do your best!

No one can do everything; that is true,
Yet the people who do all they can are so few.
You'll never know how much you can do
Unless you try what's impossible too.

Courage attempts what at first seems impossible.
Perseverance completes whatever is feasible.
Wisdom knows when you've done all you can.
Humility seeks help from your fellow man.

## TIME IS A GIFT

Time is a gift God gives us each day.
We have time to work, we have time to play,
But time, when it's lost, can never be found
Though we search for it carefully all around.
So work at work time and play at playtime,
But please remember never to waste time.
Time is a gift God gives us each day,
So use it wisely, don't throw it away. 1989


# THE RUMBLING

I was sitting in bed breast-feeding Agalia. A sudden loud noise and rumble shook the apartment building. Tracks ran parallel to our street, and we were accustomed to hearing the train. The whole building shook violently. I realized instantly that this was no train. I screamed, "Earthquake!"

Avizi, awakened by the shaking, ran from his room shrieking. In his terror, he wet his pants. I heard crashing all around the apartment. When there was a lull in the quaking, I gathered the baby in my arms and, holding on to my son, cautiously ventured toward the living room. The stackable bookshelves had tumbled right into the open space where my children would have been playing, had they been awake. The doors of the china cabinet had flown open. Several prized possessions lay shattered in the same area. I gasped in horror. In the kitchen, we had replaced the built-in ironing board with shelves for our spices. That cupboard had also spilled its contents. I tried to clean up, but couldn't do much. There had been several aftershocks, and the frightened children were clinging to me. Living on the second floor, we felt the shaking even more. My head was beginning to throb; I felt queasy and knew I was headed for a migraine.

When I turned on the radio, the news was bad. My husband had already left for work. He would not make it home for hours. No buses were running. A wall had collapsed in the garage at Cal State University, killing one student. The Whittier Narrows earthquake measured 6.1 on the Richter scale and tremors were felt throughout Los Angeles.

Then things settled down, we walked around the neighborhood. We were stunned. The rolling motion of the earth during the quake had hit one house, skipped another and kept going like that. A toppled chimney laid in one spot, a few bricks from another further along. Some houses seemed unscathed; others had walls torn from their foundations. Even our apartment building sustained some cracks. Shattered glass littered the streets.

The aftershocks were still happening days later. We all had sleep problems for months. When a passing truck sent vibrations through the building, my stomach would lurch. It felt like another earthquake and was most unsettling. Little did I know that this would mark the beginning of a season of emotional earthquakes in my life.

## *HINDSIGHT*

Red lights were flashing,
But my shortsighted vision
Couldn't read the sign.
Perfect hindsight sees
The fear of abandonment,
Its choke hold on me.

## **FIRST FAMILY VACATION**

Avizi got chicken pox just as we were planning a trip to visit some relatives in Northern California. Not wanting to infect their three-year-old cousin, we postponed our departure. Agalia remained pox-free until we arrived at the cousins' home two weeks later. To our surprise and relief, little Billy was not affected.

I packed my Tupperware cooler with fried chicken, potato salad, fruit, snacks and drinks in preparation for our first family vacation. After the car was loaded, the children and I waited impatiently for their father to leave the house. He was on the telephone. With whom? I had no clue. It was that time of the month and I was irritated at the delay. My irritation grew as I tried to cook dinner in a hot pot in our hotel room that evening. I was not getting any help with the kids. Their father kept leaving the room to do what, only God knew.

We visited the aquarium in Monterey the following day. I was more relaxed as I marveled at God's astounding creations. The children were undoubtedly having a great time. I smiled at their wide-eyed wonder as they admired the sharks, sea otters, colorful fish and other sea creatures.

The cousins welcomed us, introducing us to some of their friends. My husband turned 36 that week, so I planned a surprise birthday party. Adorned in paper hats, we ate cake and ice cream while Avizi made a speech to his dad. We tittered as Agalia, only three, tried to imitate him. Everyone seemed happy and we videotaped the occasion. I enacted a one-woman skit (costume and all) based on my Christmas poem, written in *patwa*, which was a big hit with my kids. They begged, "Say it again Mommy!"

## CHRISTMAS WITH A TROPICAL FLAVOR

When Jesus was born, angels appeared to shepherds in Bethlehem, bringing "good news of great joy...a Savior has been born...he is Christ the Lord..." (Luke 2:10-12). Imagine that angels also appeared to some Jamaican farmhands, keeping watch over their sugarcane by night. After the angels left, the farmhands said to one another, "Mek we go to Bethlehem to see dis baby de angel was talking bout, and mek we tek some sugarcane for de baby."

In this group was a man named Charlie. He was a bad man, with a foul mouth and a dirty heart. As the men ran from Jamaica to Bethlehem, Charlie was ahead of the others. The Holy Spirit confirmed the truth about the baby to Charlie, as he approached the manger. His heart was transformed. Now hear Charlie:

Who fa likle baby dat lyin' down beside de donkey?
Is dat de one de angel say would be bawn to de Virgin Mary?
Mek me go likel closer for me want to know,
If everyting de angel say is so.
Look 'pon de baby man, what a pretty likle ting!
Look how Him face ashine, Him must be really a King!
De angel say Him bring great joy and save us from our sin;
Him gwine bring us peace, and Him name is Christ De Lawd.
Christ De Lawd? Christ De Lawd! I tink I understan!
Massa God, me heart is full, dis is a wandarous sight!
You mus' really, really love us or else You know we plight.
We bawn in sin, we live in sin, and in we sin we would die,
But tonight, we have a Savior dat You sent us from on high!
Tank You, Baby Jesus, dat You care enough to come!
Massa God, tek me dirty heart, I give it to Yu beautiful son!
Clean it up and fix it up and make it fit for Dee,
Make me like a bran' new man for odder folks to see!
And afta what I see tonight, my mout' can't keep still,
I gwine tell de good news everywhere I go, I surely will! 1988

On the weekend, we visited Sequoia National Park. It truly was breathtaking. I learned that the roots of those huge redwood trees were intertwined in order to provide the support needed for each tree to stand erect. There was a lesson in that for us. I had been questioning my assumption of support from my spouse. That trust was tottering.

Avizi, just six years old and dwarfed by the enormous trees, looked up at the sky and exclaimed, "Wow! It would take me three days and three nights to climb to the top!" Who could have imagined that Avizi would say yes to his bride in the same forest, under the same gigantic trees, almost 24 years later?

# PART 4. LIBERATING JOY

## *WHO ARE YOU?*

You said I was the best thing that ever came your way,
Yet you spend so little time with me in talk or play.
You seldom laugh, never cry, and when you force a smile,
I wonder what dark secrets cower behind your cool reserve,
Or what new inexplicable outburst crouches in the gloom.
Can I shield my spirit from the debris of your next eruption?
Who is this stranger emerging with the changing of the moon?
Who strikes without warning, leaving me hurt and mystified?
I blink and stare and there you stand.
Did I not see another man? Who are you? 1988


## *WOUNDED WOLF*

You said you were a wounded wolf,
I asked you to get help,
But you refused and chose to stay
All wrapped up in yourself.

The pain, it just seemed to grow worse
And you were lashing out
Without a thought or care about
The ones who might get hurt.

I watched your wound's infection spread,
And I grew quite alarmed.
As mother-warrior it was my job
To keep the cubs from harm.

I understood to some degree
The pain that you were in,
That someone failed you as a child,
I deemed a dreadful sin.

But our two cub's protection need
Which, if you fail to give,
Leaves me no choice but to step up,
Give them a chance to live. 1990


## I WISH THEY'D WASH THEIR HANDS

Have you heard of old King Midas?
How what he touched would turn to gold?
Well there's another story like it
Which has not yet been told.

It's about two little children
Whose hands have a special touch?
Cause everything they handle
Ends up with a smear or blotch.

There is toothpaste on the ceiling,
There is mustard on the wall,
There is jelly in the bedroom,
Peanut butter in the hall.

Light switches are all gooey,
Doorknobs are sticky too,
The door of the refrigerator
Looks like it's been eating stew.

These special little children
I do love so very much!
But how I wish they'd wash their hands
Before my things they touch! 1990

# PLEASANT RECOLLECTIONS

Dear Avizi and Agalia,

Homeschooling was challenging, yet fulfilling. We enjoyed learning together, singing, dancing, reading, cooking, sewing, painting and just hanging out. On hot days we cooled our heels in the plastic pool. On cooler days, we enjoyed walking around the neighborhood, collecting pine cones, listening to the birds, and watching squirrels scamper through the trees. We baked and painted our playdough creations and watched seedlings sprout on the kitchen window. Although we often went to the park, my heart flip-flopped whenever you wandered beyond my range of vision. We laughed at Amelia Be Delia and were enthralled with the shenanigans of Roald Dahl's Matilda.

Avizi, one day you announced with pride, "Mom, I just finished reading a chapter book from Daddy's bookshelf!" That was a huge achievement for a little guy. Reading to your sister and me made you excel in that skill. You mastered all those big words so quickly! I delighted in discovering deals on books that would challenge my two voracious bookworms. Science was your favorite topic, and you read every volume of *The Book of Knowledge* encyclopedia. Your SAT scores, usually above your grade level, constantly astonished the other moms.

For your seventh birthday (the last one celebrated before your father left), we festooned the garage with balloons, colorful streamers, and the big clown we made with odds and ends from my sewing basket. Guests were impressed with your art projects on display. The kids decorated pine cones like Christmas trees. Pamela videotaped those memories for us.

Agalia, your fourth birthday, the last one celebrated with dad at home, was also recorded. We decorated with paper dolls shaped like hearts, using colored yarn for hair. The kids enjoyed singing "Agalia's Song" and playing musical chairs, while I played the accordion. Darling Debbie, an heirloom doll from your dad, was destined for destruction. Your darling brother dashed her around until she lost her head. Your other dolls all had their hair hacked off, but that was your doing.

Avizi, without reading the instructions, you assembled a desk for Agalia's room when you were only nine. I was awestruck at your dexterity. Your Lego creations were always remarkable! Remember those clown pajamas? I laid out the material; you marked and cut; I stitched. We were a great team. I still treasure the colorful, commemorative medal you made for me when I became a U.S. citizen.

When Opal and her kids came to dinner, Agalia decorated the table while you wrote out the menu. Dressed in your white shirt, you greeted our guests. "Welcome to Caribbean Café!" It was delightful to watch both of you serving our friends. Son, I had no idea then that Hospitality and Management would become your career. Daughter, who knew you would become so skilled at planning and arranging tea parties?

Whenever your dad returned home after working out of town, we displayed a "Welcome Home Dad" sign. You were always so excited to see him. Avizi, I have fond memories of the Valentine's Day you and your Daddy shopped for groceries, shut us girls out of the kitchen and prepared dinner. After decorating the kitchen with red paper hearts, you escorted Agalia and me to the table. Attired like a waiter, you read us the menu and wrote down our orders. Your dad cooked, and the meal was superb!

After dinner you asked us to remain in the kitchen until we were called. When we were allowed in the living room, paper hearts were dangling from the ceiling and music was booming from the stereo. We took turns dancing with each other. It was a happy time.

On one of my birthdays (I can't recall which one), you all banished me from the apartment. When I was invited back, your dad blindfolded and led me into the living room. You two couldn't restrain the giggles and excitement. Your father had constructed a gigantic cobweb with string. It ran helter-skelter through the apartment. My job was to follow the string and find the loot. You all kept laughing and hollering "hot" or "cold." I felt my way around, finding money taped to the cobweb. What a creative idea!

You especially loved going to the park to hang out with other homeschool families. That was where we first met Pamela and her daughter Kalen. Pamela has been a very dear friend through many years and tears. Agalia, you always hated wearing shoes. One day you took off your Buster Browns. Nobody noticed until we were almost home. We went back, but those shoes were long gone. There were so many outings and so much fun! Jasmine said Darren always begged her to homeschool him too.

The international dinner organized by our homeschool group was the last family event before your father left. Agalia, you and I wore colorful skirts and head wraps that I had made. We danced as I sang the Jamaican folk song, "This Long Time Gal." Avizi, remember how someone had to help you hop up unto the stage when, wrapped in a white sheet like an Egyptian mummy, you gave a presentation on King Tut? I still have that book you made with the Jamaican song I composed. The group really enjoyed singing it.

## JAMAICA SONG
(Tune: "Matilda")

Refrain:
Jamaica, Jamaica,
Jamaica is the land of wood and water.

Jamaica is an island;
It is surrounded by the Caribbean Sea.
White sand beaches in Montego Bay
Rafting on the Rio Grande are tings we do dere.

Banana, coconut,
Sugarcane and mango are some of the fruit we eat dere.
Cassava, duckunuh,
Chocho and gungu peas are some of the food dere.

Yellow and black and green,
Dees are de colors Jamaica's flag is made of.
Yellow is sunshine, and
Black is for de people, green for de trees and plants dere.

Arawak Indians, Africans,
Spanish and English men, dey all have lived dere.
"Out of Many One People"
Dis is de national motto of Jamaica.

Beautiful Jamaica,
It is de native country of me mada and me fada. 1990

## FRUSTRATED JOY

I believe that a healthy marriage is one in which each partner acknowledges the equality and individuality of the other. Both must also recognize the need for mutual dependence in order to achieve a healthy union. When the delicate balance of these factors is overturned, the marriage cannot be healthy. What is acceptable dependence in marriage for someone with a disability? The line often becomes blurred. Who determines what's appropriate? If my spouse is unwilling to accept my disability, he may also resent my need for him to provide necessary support. If he is insecure with an inordinate need for control, he may undermine my individuality by dictating conditions in areas that should be strictly mine to manage.

I ask him, for example, to confirm the color of panty hose I'm selecting to wear with a particular dress. Instead of answering the question, he assumes the right to order me not to wear the dress. I specifically chose that dress. I am simply borrowing his eyes, not relinquishing my ability or right to choose. I have no quarrel with him making me aware of a stain on the dress. Otherwise, insisting that I change the dress is out of order.

It isn't a matter of pleasing him; that is a normal expectation, sometimes, but his displeasure is random. His disapproval can be directed at anything — my chosen hairstyle, my daughter's hair, my shoes, clothes, or my choice to forego wearing panty hose during a heat wave. I never know what will please him. The dress was fine a week ago, but doesn't look right this week. Today, I have lovely legs and look great in shorts. Tomorrow, I will need to cover my legs because of my scars. In any case, I feel degraded when I'm backed into a corner, shunned, or treated with disdain, because I don't acquiesce to his fickle fancies.

This constant negative barrage, coupled with the subconscious voice drenching me with guilt for not submitting to my husband, distorts my personal identity. Resentment and anger increase, and my self-confidence is eroded. Few areas are left to my "undisputed" control. I no longer trust my own judgment, and dependency grows.

I do not give in easily. When I push back, my response is viewed as lack of submission. When I capitulate, it is with internal seething, which by no means implies submission. My spirit hasn't fully surrendered, but the pressure is wearing me down. I feel like something is trying to suck me up.

The fear is debilitating. I wish I didn't have to depend on him for anything, but my visual impairment is real. There are moments of intense conflict. I'm reminded of all the things he does because I can't; I am a burden; I complicate his life. How do I recover from the devastation of such declarations? Maybe our expectations of marriage were too idyllic. He now seems to feel trapped by the constraints of my disability, while I feel cheated, disillusioned by my erroneous belief that this man would fulfill my joy.

How can I be totally independent? There are times I must seek assistance from someone. If I can't depend on my husband without feeling devalued, why do I have a husband? Should I bypass him and seek help from a stranger? Does my need for help eliminate my right to make choices? Should I have a curfew imposed on the rare time spent with friends? Can I decide the menu for our daughter's birthday party without a verbal boxing match? Do I have the right to freely select an item when grocery shopping? He seems to think that asking him to assist in identifying an item translates to me asking for his permission to buy the item.

Feeling hopeless and beginning to question my sanity, I start talking to other women. They say it isn't my fault, that nothing I do will mollify his insecurities. Convinced that I am not insane, I begin to make changes with the support of friends. I can't change him, but I can alter my response to him. When I start taking certain moves toward more independence, he resists. With his power-base slipping, he attempts to exert more control. If the status quo changes, his insecurities will be exposed. He will not be able to hide behind mine.

Then one day, he was going to leave. It was a major earthquake. I was scared and did (I'm ashamed to say) cry and grovel a little. A day later, in response to my pleas, he patronizingly decided that it was in *his best interest* to stay. I was mortified!

Slowly growing stronger, I began to reverse the process of osmosis and was not going to get sucked in again. If he deserted, I would go on living, even with the pain of rejection. I knew my value. If he wanted to walk away from a person of worth, he could go, but he could not successfully blame me. I was not asking him to leave. The children were my greatest concern. How would I protect them from the hurt?

I am reclaiming my personal power, but the marriage is still far from healthy. When, momentarily, inhibitions are abandoned and some intimacy is achieved, it is soon undermined by passive-aggressive action. I am therefore wary and afraid of becoming too relaxed. Perfect love removes fear, but fear corrodes love.

An insightful person said that anyone who denies his own insecurities can never be rid of them. Driven by subconscious forces, he will attack and destroy anyone who threatens his illusion of security and power. Understanding this, I remain very troubled concerning my mental and emotional health in our marriage. Action fueled by fear and anger cannot nurture love and trust. Wisdom dictates certain independent moves for the guarantee of my emotional well-being and personal power over my own life.

How do I reconcile my need for independence with the vulnerabilities presented by my visual impairment? Fear must be dispelled. How can it be when my spouse's behavior and disparaging utterances undermine my self-confidence? Only God has the answer.

I wish He'd give it to me. My spouse and I have come to a crossroads. Do we travel on together, or do we part? I wish to go on, to salvage the marriage, but do not intend to maintain the status quo. How do I resolve this conflict? Can it be resolved?

I believe that submission and authority are part of God's blueprint for marriage, but I wrestle with their practical application. Outward submission is of no value to God if the heart does not participate. My heart cannot participate if the submission demanded is a violation of my God-affirmed personhood and equality. I know my sinful nature sometimes resists appropriate submission. Only the Holy Spirit can help me discern the one from the other, and enable me to submit as God requires. I seek this understanding.

I desire to love without fear. I want to be able to entrust my person to the man who vowed before God to nourish and cherish me. These are the outpourings of a frustrated woman. (May, 1990)

"Who can discern his errors? Forgive my hidden faults. Keep your servant also from willful sins; may they not rule over me. Then will I be blameless, innocent of great transgression. May the words of my mouth and the meditations of my heart be pleasing in your sight, O Lord, my Rock and my Redeemer." Psalm 19:12-14

## *PILGRIMAGE OF A SURVIVOR*

I've been told I'm no good and would come to no good,
I've been sinned against, blamed and misunderstood.
My heart screamed in defense as if it would burst,
But no one could hear so I lived with the curse.
I gave up the protest, bought into the lie
Which has kept me prisoner for much of my life.
Though a prisoner, I struggled, I had to survive.
So in my dreams nightly the protest revived.

Though to many around I was always achieving,
None knew of the guilt and the shame I was feeling.
I banished the truth while I locked in the lie,
Living in pain, sometimes wanting to die.
I was looking for love in some unsafe places,
Putting my trust in some unsafe faces.
In searching for love, I lowered my standards.
For fool's gold, my worth and my dignity squandered.

Some that I trusted have caused me much pain,
Leaving me feeling that I was to blame.
I didn't fight back for it had been foretold.
What happened to me did the first lie uphold.
Guilt I carried for years like a weight on my back.
Chastising, accusing, he gave me no slack.
With this constant annoying companion
All residual feelings of worth were abandoned.

I had heard that God loved me, I believed in His Son,
I confessed all the wrong things I knew I had done.
Yet, I couldn't stop feeling the guilt and the shame.
I lived in great torment, myself I still blamed.
Others had hurt me, put on me their wrong,
I felt responsible for what they had done.
Bad things do not happen to those who are good,
So, I must be bad…that's what I understood.

For survival, I froze, though I was not quite dead.
I knew that God loved me, but just in my head.
The truth of His Love had not penetrated
The emotional iceberg which I had created.
I felt so unworthy, some folks reinforced it.
I tried hard to please so I would be accepted.
I struggled for freedom while some held me back,
Trying to control me for power they lacked.

For things I accomplished I had been applauded
Yet, deep in my heart I did not feel rewarded.
I labored in torment, with deep-seated fear.
If I did not succeed, no love would be there.
This state of affairs went on for years.
I spent many nights shedding copious tears.
Despite heart-wounds and thinking that's twisted,
Complete defeat I strongly resisted.

Something within me fought for survival
And slowly but surely, began a revival.
Change had to come, I could stay down no more!
Something within me was starting to soar.
For long, I had earnestly searched for the truth,
Somewhere within me was planted a root.
Struggling through all the morass and the slime
Of my screwed-up emotions, it started to climb.

As it surfaced in freedom from the muck and the mire,
It gathered momentum climbing higher and higher!
As I reached out for truth, The Truth embraced me
And, as Jesus had promised, I began to be free!
I'm discarding the lies, I believe what God said,
The process of healing has begun in my head.
I can grow and glow, even fail yet go on
For I know my God loves me without condition.

I saw how God loved me, had called me by name,
Had sent His Son Jesus to bear all my shame.
I saw He had wept when others had hurt me,
I saw He had patiently waited to heal me.
I discovered the gifts God had lavished on me,
What He'd done to establish my own dignity.
I arose and reclaimed my personal power.
Now my strength is increasing hour by hour!

I can love myself because God loved me first,
Assigning my potential before my birth.
He had cared all those years when I lived in such pain.
Not once did He ever forget my name!
Lord, thanks for relieving the weight of my burden,
For soothing and healing the wounds I was nursing,
For strength to forgive those who have sinned against me,
For hearing my prayer and setting me free.

Keep my mind clear, for the battle goes on.
When I do right, I still sometimes feel wrong.
Help me go forward, whatever the cost,
Believing that, with You, the battle is not lost.
May I not falter in doing what's good,
Renew me and help me to walk as I should.
Strengthen my faith, my mind, my body,
As I endeavor to do my duty.

Teach me to love me as much as You do,
To seek fulfillment only in You.
Then, when I'm filled up with true joy and peace,
To others these gifts I can freely release.
For how can I properly love my neighbor
If I have not learned to accept the Lord's favor?
If I shut out Your Love, I have naught to give others,
If I don't first receive, I can't give to my brothers.

Teach me to show myself compassion,
To tend my own needs without reservation,
To use the same energy in caring for me
That I waste on those I am trying to please.
I need not give all when others I help,
A cupful of mercy I can pour on myself,
I need not say yes to all the demands,
I am free to say no or to change my plans.

I can throw out self-doubt and incompetence;
I don't have to be weak or deny my good sense.
I can rock the boat if I think it needs rocking,
I can speak the truth though it might be quite shocking!
I can think my own thoughts and act my own act
And with nobody's permission, at that!
I can take what is mine, what I need, I need.
Who I am, I am! I'm not here just to please!

Lord, sometimes I do and sometimes I doubt,
Take my unbelief, help me work it out.
After forty-two years, it's not easy to change
A life of self-doubt, self-rejection and blame.
Teach me right now how to lean hard on You,
Exposing the lies, believing what's true,
Then finally, help me to understand
That I dare not put my trust in man. 1990

"Blessed is he whose help is in the God of Jacob, whose hope is in the Lord his God, the Maker of heaven and earth...who remains faithful forever." Psalm 146:5, 6.

## PARADOX

People, they're a paradox;
I just can't understand them.
They can make you; they can break you;
They can love you; they can hate you.
People, they're a paradox;
I just can't understand them! 1972

## NO VOICE

Children must be seen, not heard, so I lost my voice;
Frightened, I said nothing, didn't think I had a choice.
Perpetrators did their thing, put the blame on me,
I bought the lie they told me, for the truth I couldn't see.
Suffering in silence to maintain the status quo,
I remained a victim, too scared to tell them no.
Now I forgive my elders for taking away my voice,
For heartaches I endured when I was left without a choice.


## BETRAYAL

When I was born they called me Joy,
As I grew up you doted on me.
Because I thought you truly cared,
I felt encouraged that you were there.

My own dad was so critical,
He put me down at every turn,
He made me feel I had no worth,
My heart for validation yearned.

When you were good and kind to me,
My thirsty soul just drank it up;
When you were bad, shock and dismay
Left me with no words to say.

I had you on a pedestal
So I put myself beneath its base,
I thought it true what Dad had said,
I really wasn't any good.

For years you robbed me of my joy,
For years I lived a silent hell.

Those years have gone and I have grown
To understand you did me wrong.

"Why bring it up? It's been so long.
Forgive, forget," I hear you say,
But to forgive I must go back
And clarify the harm you've done.

Denial never changes truth
And garbage covered up just festers,
So I must call a spade a spade,
Dig up the sordid thoughts that pester.

It's time for you to take the stand,
Before God you're a guilty man.
Whether you own it or deny,
Joy must purge herself of lies.

No more am I a timid girl
Afraid to stand up to her elders,
I'll not carry your guilt and shame,
I'm putting back on you your pain! 1992

"It is better to take refuge in the Lord than to trust in man."
Psalm 118:8


## WHO'S A SLAVE?

He's a slave, the man who taunts his woman
With verbal and emotional degradations,
Who derides her when she dares to dream,
By saying how stupid and foolish it seems.

If she maintains her strength and masters her plan,
So little is he, so unlike a real man
That he hastens to steal her compliments
And basks in the glory of her achievements.

He's a slave, the man who with jealousy seethes
At every success that his wife achieves.
He can never applaud her for getting ahead
But muddles her thinking with mind games instead.

He's a slave, the man who can never rest
But must prove to the world and himself he's the best.
He rarely spends time with his family,
He's so busy conquering the earth, you see.

There's no job he can't handle, no hill he won't climb
Trying to solve all the social ills of his time.
He will face any challenge except his own
And forgets that charity begins at home.

His home life's a mess and he's aching inside,
Yet his secrets and shame he'll to no one confide,
He puts on a big show and lies to himself
But the truth, if exposed, would the lie soon dispel.

He's a slave, the man who already knows
His check can't support his family and his clothes.
He insists on spending beyond his means
While his wife and kids wear tattered old jeans.

He is haughty and proud and how he can brag!
It's surprising he ever removes the price tags.
He looks down at his wife and makes a grimace:
"Too short, too fat, nose too big, mars my image!"

He's a slave, the man who must have his liquor
To keep himself in perpetual stupor,
Who numbs the pain that gnaws at his soul
Then bullies and batters the wife he controls.

He's a slave, the man whose lust must be fed,
Who wants to be in every woman's bed.
He calls it a conquest each time he does it,
But who is really conquered, can you guess it?

Slavery has been abolished so long
And still I hear this same sad song:
"A man's gotta have!" No! A man's gotta BE!
Be a real man if you want to be free!

Let God break the fetters that imprison your soul.
He'll grant you forgiveness and make you whole.
Deal in truth, stop believing the lie.
Own your pain, look yourself in the eye.

You thought wielding your power would make you feel good?
You believed the lie for you never understood
That he who shackles and breaks another's soul
Is himself in shackles and not in control.

Lynch the lie, learn the truth and then you'll see
That only truth can set a man free.
Be a slave no more, turn the light on your pain,
When the darkness flees there'll be so much to gain!

Become the man you were ordained to be
By God, not by corrupt society.
Cry to the Lord for the freedom you need,
Ask Him to set your Black soul free.

Own the pain, break the chain, then Jesus will give
Freedom to live and let others live,
Freedom to dream and stretch and climb
And reach your potential in your own time!

Rise up, Black men! Be free! Be strong!
Be the men your women can safely lean on.
We've been yearning and longing to see you "free
At last," the men God ordained you to be. 1990

"I tell you the truth, everyone who sins is a slave to sin...if the Son sets you free, you will be free indeed." John 8:34, 36

## *TURN ME LOOSE!*

This caged bird just won't sing
If you don't set me free to exercise my wings.
Clip my wings and you clip your joy,
'Cause I'm not a child and I'm not a toy!
I'm an independent spirit with needs and ambitions
And I can't survive under these conditions.

Cage me up too long, and when the moment comes
For you to open the door, I'll already be gone.
I can be here and gone—you catch the drift?
So when I ask for freedom, don't you resist!
I'm not a child nor a toy, you see,
But a grown-up with equal rights—that's me!

Now I don't ask for much, don't just ask for me,
'Cause the children will benefit ultimately,
But it seems that you would sacrifice them too
So you can be free to do what you want to do.
You have the power to stay or leave
Just about any time you please.

Well, some of that power is mine to share,
Though where I'm concerned there is no scare.
I don't plan to go 'cause I know commitment
Though I find myself in this grave predicament.
So turn me loose and let me stretch my wings
Or you'll never hear this caged bird sing!

Now I'm not saying I'll never sing,
But you will miss the joy my song can bring.
I will sing for folks who want to see me free.
I won't sing for folks who imprison me.
So turn me loose and let me stretch my wings
Or you'll never hear this caged bird sing!

I've got to have time off, you see,
If I'm to flourish and bloom creatively.
I need fresh air and I need the sun,
I need to revitalize my song.
I need a chance to soar, the sky to fly,
Or in this stifling cage I'll shrivel and die.

Turn me loose and I'll come back to you,
It's the best thing you could ever do,
Just turn me loose to aim for the sky
Then sit right back and watch me fly.
As I spread my wings you will hear me sing
From the pure, sheer joy that freedom brings!

I must sing my song till my journey's done,
Till the Good Lord comes to carry me home.
So open the door and get out of the way,
In this cage I can no longer stay.
And if you try to smother or hold me down,
You'll never, never, hear my song! 1990

## SHOP IS SHUT!

I don't want to do business with folk who disrespect me or my property, who don't know what they want. They come in here, high and mighty, trying to put their confusion on me. I just won't stand for it! I have done too much to get this far for folk to mess with my head or play havoc with my spirit. I have no particular urge to visit the funny farm, so I'm closing down! I'm boarding up!

No use beating down the door. Can't you read? The sign says, *"Shop is Shut!"* Don't you try to sweet-talk me now. I've had enough of that! I'll reopen when I've reworked the store with burglar-bars on windows and doors. Then, I'll decide if I want to let you in. And if I do, my treasures will be in full view but out of reach. The *"DO NOT TOUCH"* sign hanging overhead will not come down till you display a new appreciation for my wares, some gesture of remorse for things destroyed. But if you trifle with me, or make one negative remark about my store's arrangement, I'll have you thrown out hard upon your head, and that will be for good!

Perhaps, if shop stays shut, you will recall the ease with which you sauntered in and out my store, from the shelves snatching whatever you wanted, and out the door striding without even paying. Perhaps you'll recall merchandise you nonchalantly dropped, careless of their fragility, unappreciative of their value. Perhaps you'll remember cries of dismay, tears mingling with the mess you made, the smirk on your face as you strolled out the door, satisfied you'd scored again. The opportunity to trade, at last denied, may cause my gems to gather value in your eyes. And when again I open shop, perhaps you'll have a new respect for who I am and what I've got.
1990

# CLOSED FOR SPRING CLEANING

I gave you the key, let you into my spirit,
Which you vandalized in a merciless manner.
What I, like a fool, gave to you on a platter,
You've spat out and, with contempt, thrown away.

"I'm sorry" rolled glibly off of your tongue
Each time that my spirit lay battered and bruised.
You could say such soothing and penitent words
Whenever I wept from your mental abuse.

I believed against reason, showed you forgiveness,
Then you'd start the head trips and mind games again;
While I went on dreaming the dream of the foolish,
The cycle repeated each time as before.

My spirit is closed now for some renovating.
To your moods and whims I am no longer catering.
My mind is shut up, I've exhausted endurance,
My rights as a person I'm now reasserting.

No promise you make now, however alluring,
Will comfort this fool or muddle her head.
I'll unravel the webs that entangle my thinking,
Delete thoughts that cripple, toss dreams that are dead.

I'll unlock the closet, let out the feelings
That have been stuffed there for such a long time.
I'll brush the dust from my album of memories
While slowly retracing the hills I have climbed.

I will clear the clutter, throw out all the garbage,
Remove the confusion that's long settled here.
I'll give the old attic a new coat of fresh paint,
Let in clean air for what's dying in there.

My spirit is closed now but just for a season.
I'll throw open the window with gusto again.
I'll hang up new curtains, I'll live like it's springtime,
Dismissing the doldrums of winter's pain.

I'll sing with the birds, I'll dance as the raindrops
Wash all the grime from my window panes.
I'll look back of the clouds for a new silver lining,
Turn my eyes to the hills with hope once again.

For my Helper knows how to give beauty for ashes.
How well He knows how to bring joy out of pain!
So when I am done counting all of my losses,
I'll trust Him to turn them all into gain. 1991

# PART 5. JOY ON THE ROCKS

## STRANGER THAN FICTION

I had a dream. The children and I were wandering on the street looking for their father. It was nighttime and we couldn't find our way home. I awoke, alarmed. I had another dream a few weeks later. This time, the four of us stood in an open field. In the distance was a huge warehouse. As we watched, two men emerged from the building pushing an empty shopping cart toward us. One of them held a large syringe. He jabbed the needle into my spouse's arm. I stared in horror as he collapsed. Without a word, the men hoisted him into the cart and headed for the warehouse. Stunned and speechless, I stood riveted to the spot, until they disappeared. The dream ended.

I don't really know what to call the experience I had a few months later. Returning home from a recovery group meeting in deep emotional pain, I headed for the bedroom. It was 8:00 PM. My spouse was in the kitchen. The lights were on. I laid on the far side of the bed away from the door.

Suddenly, I saw my husband slowly moving around the bed. As he drew closer, he seemed more sinister. Terrified, I began to struggle, in the grip of some evil force. In this state, call it a trance, vision or dream, I know not what, I tried to say the name of Jesus. I couldn't get it out. The force broke abruptly. I heard myself cry out. I wasn't sure what I said, but the sound of my voice brought me out of whatever that was. My spouse came running from the kitchen.

"Are you okay? I heard you calling for your mother!" Still in a daze, I stared at him before responding.

"Are you planning to hurt me again?" Walking away, he muttered, in apparent confusion, "What are you talking about?"

# TURNING POINT

When my spouse first threatened to leave, then decided it was in *his best interest* to stay, a wise woman advised me to make changes in preparation for when it would no longer be in *his best interest*. She also encouraged me to "strive to be better, not bitter." Neither suggestion was easy.

Years before, I had heard recently widowed women on a radio program, discussing the shock of being totally in the dark regarding their finances. I determined then that it wouldn't happen to me. Voicing my concerns, I started managing our money. For the next year, amid subversive tactics, I worked at improving our finances. In the process, I discovered how to use credit cards to my advantage, not to help some CEO purchase another yacht.

To reduce excessive fees, I changed banks. Borrowing money from my father, I consolidated and eliminated credit card debt. Daddy had his money back in a year, and we had a nest egg of $400. When I opened my first credit card account—in my name only—my partner queried about my credit limit. With an air of superiority, he disclosed how much higher his limit was (as if plastic money is real money). I had cleared and closed several accounts when, demonstrating his financial laxity, he opened a new account with an annual fee.

"If we have so little money to show for all our years of marriage, why don't you get a card with no annual fee like the average person?" I offered an idea for further enhancing our fiscal health. He ignored me. The next day, I was washing dishes when he approached me. "I have an idea. Why don't we…?" He repeated my previously ignored idea as if it were his own. I looked at him, incredulous. Without a word, I scrubbed the dishes with greater fervor. It was a game and I was done playing.

One day, he blurted out, "I know I have to get my act together because I know you understand the concept of tough love." I was surprised. A window of truth was suddenly opened, but was slammed shut just as quickly. I looked at him, but said nothing. Weary of talking, I had been reading James Dobson's *Love Must Be Tough*. I had also read *Codependent No More* by Melody Beattie. Trying to recover from the "disease to please," I was setting new boundaries.

Disheartened by our pastor's flippant response to our problems, I contacted a counselor regarding an intervention. The date was set after soliciting the participation of some mutual *friends*. I believe strongly that one of them tipped him off.

Two days before my 43$^{rd}$ birthday and one month past our 11$^{th}$ anniversary, my husband called me into the bedroom to talk. That was the first shock. He wanted to talk. He would be leaving in four days. Instead of treating myself to dinner on my birthday, I bought a *good* vacuum cleaner with a portion of the savings and started cleaning. That was a wholesome outlet for my anger. Two days later, as promised, my spouse took his clothing and departed.

Systematically, I removed papers from his file cabinet, stacked them in boxes, labeled the boxes, and put his remaining belongings in the garage. Guarding against possible harassment, I asked the landlord to change the locks. I would not be disrespected in my grief. My message was clear the next time he tried to open the door. In compromising our covenant, he had abdicated his authority as head of this household. His right to enter my home at will had been forfeited; his power to issue orders—null and void! I didn't beg him to stay and I didn't cry, at least not in his presence.

That summer, the children and I left for Boston. Their father called frequently, saying he missed his family and wanted to change. When we returned home some months later, nothing changed. For the next few years, we did a deadly dance that almost made me crazy, but we never lived together again. I have heard stories of women who made that mistake to their own detriment.

Overwhelmed by the pain of rejection, I lost my joy. Knowing the children needed me, I started taking an antidepressant to help me cope. With support from a counselor, and the resolve to profit from pain, I became stronger. I continued to turn up the heat on my prodigal spouse. The counselor advised me to keep my boundaries in place whether he was "naughty or nice."

After several disingenuous attempts at reconciliation, my spouse announced his plan to divorce me based on irreconcilable differences. It was the weekend before Mother's Day. Although I had been slowly unraveling the web of our enmeshment, the announcement stung. I didn't understand why God had not saved my marriage. Didn't He say He hates divorce (Malachi 2:16)? I recalled my friend's injunction to be better, not bitter. That was going to be very hard!

"So you are abandoning your family for real."

"I have never failed my children as a father. I am not leaving them, just you."

"Really! Is that what you plan to tell them?"

## SHATTERED JOY

I sat you both upon my knees,
Told you Daddy was going to leave.
Fat tears came rolling down your face,
Your pain I knew I couldn't erase.
"How will we get to Sunday school?
Will Dad take his Legos too?"
I had no answer for you then,
I knew not how we three would fend.
My pain intensified by yours
Within my heart a deep hole bored.
I saw and felt the shattered joy
Of my little girl and boy.

## LIFE IS NOT PERFECT

Life is like a dungeon
When everything goes wrong.
Count on God the Father
To help us all be strong.

God will help us do good things
If we always trust in Him.
We will win the battle strong
Even if the fight is long.
If we have faith in the Lord,
We will take Him at His Word.
So if we confess our sins
He will give us righteousness.
(By Avizi & Agalia, 1991)


## FROM THE MOUTHS OF BABES

Avizi, you were eight years old and your sister just five when your Daddy left. The times you both played with those tiny Lego bricks were very special, and you wondered if they would leave with him too. Difficult days followed, but, with God's help, we plodded on. When we went shopping (mostly for you kids) and stopped for lunch, there was never enough money for all of us. I bought you and your sister what you wanted, then took a bite from each of you.

One day, we went shopping with Sandra and her kids. I found a dress I really liked. At the checkout, I was ambivalent about the purchase. Observing my hesitation, Sandra encouraged, "Buy the dress, you deserve it!" My son, you astonished me when you exclaimed, "It's about time!" I had no idea you had been paying such close attention. Your comment warmed my heart. I bought the dress!

At our new church, Pastor Jim was preaching about trials. He said God only sends trials to someone who can handle them. If you are chosen, it means you are special and just need to hold on. I was touched when you whispered, "That's for you, Mom!" You were not quite nine years old, yet you understood that Mom was hurting.

# VIRTUAL BODY BAG

They say good things come in small packages, but this was big! A monstrosity! A great big body bag was shoved in my face. It created such panic within me, I could not touch or examine it for some time. The deliverer of this ominous package presented it with a speech that went like this: "I will never be the person you want me to be. You are a good woman with a lot of gifts. You will do better without me. Head for the sun."

"So you are choosing the darkness?" It was a rhetorical question. For the next three months, working around this omen of death, so suddenly projected into the center of my existence, I ran myself ragged in an effort to evade the inevitable. Needing to do anything but contemplate the contents of the dreaded bag, I discarded old furniture and junk. I haggled with the landlord for a fresh coat of paint and new carpet. When there was nothing else to clean, I took a vacation with the children.

There was no escaping. I had to return home and confront my new reality. It was finally time to delve into my undesirable present. As I unzipped the bag and began removing the packaging, I realized why I had been so afraid of this task.

Piece by piece, I pulled out the excess baggage: anger, resentment, insecurity, guilt, blame, shame, failure, rejection, fear...so much pain and fear! I had to stop. Filled with a plethora of conflicting emotions, I threw myself in an exhausted heap on a makeshift bed in the corner, unable to sleep in the master bedroom.

Not at all liking its contents, I pursued the task of emptying this gift bag. For weeks, I unearthed more conflict, pain and tears, not finding anything of value. Several friends observed that I looked as if a load had rolled off my shoulders. I thought they were just trying to make me feel good. The pain was so intense, I felt like crawling into that body bag and zipping it up around me. Reluctantly, I continued to exhume its contents.

Suddenly one morning, I grasped something firm. Unwrapping it cautiously, I found new enlightenment. I was stunned. In my hand was a precious jewel! Then, for the first time, I noticed the sunlight streaming in through the windows. Surrounded by all this light, I recognized that freedom was in my hand. It was in my hand! How could this be? My broken heart was real. Pain was real. This treasure in my hand was also real. I was momentarily bewildered. What would I do with it? That was now my decision.

Among the wretchedness of the excess baggage left me by my fleeing spouse, was a gift of incomparable value. I was free; free to grant myself the time and space needed to mend my broken heart; free to grieve without taunting or minimization. In weakness, I had not sufficiently valued this gem God had long before bestowed on me. My mate, in turn, had not valued me. I was now free to pursue God's pure love, rather than the tainted love of a man too broken to give or receive joy. He had run from me to embrace an illusion. Through God's grace, I have even made the choice to forgive him.

Had I not chosen to face my new reality, I would never have discovered the pearl of personal freedom. I faced the truth and it has set me free. The day my body bag was delivered, I also presented my departing spouse with a gift: *Healing the Masculine Soul* by Gordon Dalby. I don't know if he ever opened his gift.

## FREEDOM

I opened my eyes in the morning
To the light streaming in through the blinds,
Symbolic not just of the morning
But the awakening of a free mind.

I once was entombed in a dungeon
Where the darkness had entered my brain,
My dreams were gradually vanishing
Like a rapidly moving train.

I struggled for sunlight and freedom,
But some powerful chains held me down,
Till I learned how to break chains asunder
With truth to which my mind still clung.

My partner, too chained in the darkness,
Had grown cynical, bitter and scared;
He hampered my progress toward freedom,
Alarmed that I'd leave him there.

For a while I relinquished my struggles
To rescue him from misery;
I spent half my strength trying to free him,
But a prisoner he wanted to be.

With the strength that remained I continued
Striving for liberty.
Determination slowly rekindled
The dying embers in me.

I had almost severed the last links.
My opponent was selfish and cold.
He tried subtle ways to restrain me,
Afraid to relinquish control.

Then an incredibly transforming thing happened,
And I knew at last I was free.
My mate had embraced new captivity
And was no longer fighting with me.

I awoke one morning to realize
That I was alone in my cell
Which had been by a miracle transformed
And I was doing quite well.

Was this just a long night and bad dream?
Have I recovered from insanity?
Did I imagine my torment?
Was my imprisonment real?

It was real for the wounds I'm still nursing

And my heart is still bloody and scarred,
But the thrill of the freedom I've found now
Dwells together with pain in my heart.

I will never again let another
Imprison me in his own hell,
I will treasure me for I'm special,
I will never abandon myself.

If my spouse wants to join my new ventures,
He must first his captivity leave,
For I will go backwards for no one
And I'm moving ahead with great speed.

If we do not strive against darkness,
It will in time put out the light,
And in chains we'll remain forever
If we have no courage to fight. 1991

While reading *Women Who Love Too Much* by Robin Norwood, I discovered a truth that sent shock waves through my body and soul. The fact is, my deep-seated neediness and fear of being alone led to fruitless efforts. I could not love my spouse enough for him to love me back. In trying, I tolerated unacceptable behavior for far too long. When this truth hit me, I wailed! The thing I feared most had happened. I sobbed with reproaches against myself for all the wasted energy. My crying was a cleansing, denial done.

I had made my husband an idol, robbing God of time and devotion that belonged only to Him. I had been afraid of being alone. Was I really alone? No! In that moment, God offered me forgiveness for my foolish, manipulative behavior and renewed His promises to love me always (Psalm 32:1-11). Such assurance brought me solace and strength to trust when I couldn't see my way.

"It is for freedom that Christ has set you free. Stand firm, then, and do not let yourselves be burdened again by a yoke of slavery." Galatians 5:1

## MERCY

I see my Savior bending low
And on His face compassion shows.
He's come to hold you in your pain,
To bring you healing once again.

I see Him gently wipe your tears,
I hear Him soothing all your fears:
"For this very thing I came,
To take away your guilt and shame.

The enemy has tried to ruin
The work that I began in you;
He's found your vulnerable parts
And shot you full of fiery darts.

You hurt, I know, that's why I'm here
To let you know that I still care.
Those darts I once felt in my side
And with your pain identify.

My love is strongest when you're weak.
Safe vigil I'll around you keep,
Till on your feet you'll stand again
And proclaim My mercy to all men." 1991

## THE PRODIGAL'S CALL

My child, you are Mine, I've called you by name,
And My love for you is always the same.
Though others have hurt you and filled you with pain,
Though you are broken, My love still remains.
You've turned on yourself, not knowing your worth,
You've been running in circles inflicting much hurt
On the ones that I gave you to love and protect.
You've been so self-centered, their needs you neglect.

I've been waiting so long, hoping you'd come
To receive My forgiveness for what you have done.
The wife of your youth has besought me with tears
To release you from bondage that's grown through the years.
She's asked me to let you see your behavior
And then from them to be your Savior,
To rescue you from destructive self-hate,
To break your bad habits before it's too late.

Your wife's fervent prayers cannot go unheeded,
In faith and in love she has long interceded.
What she asks for you is what I have wanted,
For my desires I've in her heart planted.
She once was like you, also running from pain,
But found out that running would bring her no gain.
I give her my strength as the truth she pursues,
That's how she knows I can do it for you.

Because I am God, I accomplish My will.
Because I am God, I am loving you still.
Because I am God, I can heal and restore,
No matter how hopeless life seemed before.
Because I am God, I can break and remake,
Bring beauty from ashes, remold and reshape
Any life that's entrusted to My love and care,
That is why, precious child, I've been waiting right here.

Come home, for I've started a good work in you.
Come home with My promise to see you through.
Turn away from the dark, let the light of the sun
Be a guide to your steps till My will you have done.
I'm your Daddy, I'll never abandon nor leave you,
I'll always be here, I have so much to give you!
I'll show you how to be My kind of man,
Then you can do the same for your son.

There's a void in your daughter her mother can't fill,
She's hurting inside, yet she prays for you still.
Don't leave her sad heart to wander for years,
Come home and make good with repentance and tears.
Come home and restore your family's joy,
Come show a real man to that girl and boy.
Let other men know there is hope, for I Am,
That restoration and healing are in My plan. 1991

## THE WOUNDED CHILD INSIDE YOU

There is a wounded child inside you who was hurt and abandoned in the past. He is cringing in the shadows, weeping in despair, wide-eyed with terror and fear. He is waiting, longing for someone to embrace him in love and tenderness. He feels sad and alone, believing no one can ever love him. Though full of hurt, his eyes retain a spark of hope that you might be the one to rescue him. Will you embrace him? Can you see his pain and walk away?

Abandon him no more! Embrace him! Tell him he is worthy. Tell him you will never run from him again. Tell him you will carry him from the darkness into the light, shielding his eyes with your big hands until he grows accustomed to it. Tell him he has promise and potential for good, that there are others who want to love him.

Bring him home so we can love him too. He needs a commitment from you so he can grow, come out of hiding and not be afraid. Tell him he is a worthy soul for whom Christ died. If you abandon him, he will lose all hope. Give him love so he will have love to give. Give him hope that God can heal his pain. Give him a dream of a better tomorrow, surrounded by those who genuinely care. Give him strength to go on by your commitment to stand with him even in moments of weakness. Tell him you will be there always.

# CARPET CLEANING FIASCO

Have you ever responded to those carpet cleaning ads that come in your mailbox? You know, the ones that offer to clean your carpet for $20? Well, the last time I did that was the last time I did that. The carpet cleaner from the abyss entered my life shortly after my husband had exited. A large, burly man arrived with his assistant and began to demonstrate his product. After cleaning a small area in the living room, he started his sales pitch, trying to convince me to pay $159 for a more thorough job. I told him I only had $20, so he generously offered to drive me to the bank. When I said there was no money in the bank, he resourcefully offered to put it on *my* credit card. I declined. He became agitated and registered his displeasure with loud and increasingly venomous language. To calm him down, or so I thought, I gently touched his arm and said, "Please, just do what the $20 will cover."

The man let out a tirade of expletives, accusing me of physically abusing him. He immediately called his boss to log a complaint. The boss, apparently a less than ethical person, threatened to call the police.

"What's going on up there?" My neighbor, Susan, heard the commotion and was concerned. The culprit grabbed his equipment and stormed down the stairs. His assistant, a quiet young man, watched from the background.

"I am really sorry," the young man whispered at the security gate as the offender packed up his gear. "This is my first day on the job and I wanted to jump out of the truck. I think the man is nuts. On the way here he was swearing and weaving in and out of traffic like a drunk."

Terrified and almost in tears, I explained to my neighbor what had happened. It felt as if I had been mauled by a wild animal. I felt violated and vulnerable. I was so shaken! It took days for the raw pain to subside even a little. The woman who answered the phone at the police station assured me that no one had called. She empathized and advised that I never let anyone into my house again, unless they were from a reputable company.

When I went to service my vacuum cleaner later that day, I inquired about the cost of a carpet shampooer. For the same amount that crazy man had tried to extort, I purchased a small carpet cleaner, charging it to my credit card. That evening, the young man I mentioned earlier showed up at my back door with his wife. I was surprised to see him and more amazed at what he divulged.

"After we left, he went to the phone on the corner yelling and raging as he talked to the boss. I was so scared, I jumped out of the truck when he wasn't looking, and ran into the dry cleaner's on the corner. I asked them if I could hide until he was gone. This was my first day on the job, and my last. You are the one who was abused. I am really sorry for what happened to you."

The fact that this young man came back to apologize reminded me that there were still decent people in the world. He really did not need to apologize for anything. In fact, I believe his presence may have saved me from further mistreatment. I now do my own cleaning. That carpet cleaner can just go back where he came from.

## DECEIVED

I once fell prey to a certain delusion,
That was when all the trouble began.
I had a strong need to create an illusion
Of an honest protective man.

You called me naive and you had good reason,
You alone knew the games that you played.
I loved you but now you've committed high treason,
Of my trust a mockery made.

The illusion has ended, the mirage has receded,
The rug has been yanked out from under my feet.
I'm dazed and bewildered for I was deceived
And I'm no longer sure what is real. 1993

## *DON'T YOU KNOW YOU ARE AN EAGLE?*

Don't you know that an eagle wasn't made for the ground?
Then why are you hanging around
With earth-bound turkeys going nowhere,
Held back by the weight of their own fat flesh,
In their smugness unaware
That those who fatten them today
Will later slaughter and devour?
Why work so hard for the "Turkey of the Year" award?

Have you ever seen chickens headed for the sky?
No, no, they'll never fly!
From the coop to the table is all they are able
In their very short lives.
Then why live like a chicken just a-greedily pecking
At the infested corn
Tossed you by the world?
Why work so hard for the "Chicken of the Year" award?

Don't you know you're an eagle who was born to fly high?
Then why hover around on such barren ground
With stunted birds headed nowhere?

Aren't you aware that you were meant to soar
Far above the common crowd,
Destined to reach for more
Even past the darkest cloud
Where neither chickens nor turkeys can go?

Come spread your eagle wings, reach for the sky,
Stretching your vision beyond the horizon.
Fill your lungs with clean, fresh air,
Feel the thrill of a new life;
Don't look back or down, just look ahead!
Leave behind the wrong you've done,
Keep your face toward the sun,
Shed the weight that's held you down and come on home.


## COME FOR ME

For years I have waited
While indecisive, you have loitered
In the territory of my heart,
Indifferent to the suffering you've inflicted,
Conflicted about the love you have resisted,
Filling your reservoir by draining mine.
I am tired now,
Tired of being put on hold,
Tired of being left in the cold.
That you are present yet aloof
Is insufficient proof
Of your caring for or wanting me.
Do not linger any longer
If you'll not embrace my pain!
Being committed to non-commitment
Brings me no gain!
If you do not love me, let me go,
If you've found another, tell me so.

But if you choose me, bring commitment!
Do not just come for marriage, come for me!


## THE EMPTY COKE MACHINE

I put my quarter in with ease
The way I was supposed to.
I did the proper sequences
The way I had been taught.
I reached my hand out eagerly
For I was getting thirsty,
But no Coke came out to quench my thirst.

I tried again with patient care,
Perhaps I'd made an error.
I gently put a quarter in
And firmly pressed the lever.
Again I stretched my hand out,
My thirst was getting greater,
But no Coke came out to quench my thirst.

With confidence I tried again,
It had to work the third time.
I watched as others sipped their Cokes,
Sure I'd soon be sipping mine.
My lips were chapped and parched now
So I tried again a fourth time,
But still no Coke came out to quench my thirst.

My patience now was running thin,
I grimaced and I grumbled,
I glared and then I glowered
At the screwed-up Coke machine.

My anger, it changed nothing,
For the Coke machine just stood there,
Unable or unwilling to produce.

Feeling dumb as people watched me,
I walked away exhausted.
I'd come back and try tomorrow
Maybe dressed a different way.
If I could smile more sweetly,
Place the quarter more discreetly,
Then the Coke machine will give me what I need.

I put the quarter in next day,
My luck was not improving.
Why couldn't I get a Coke
From this confounded Coke machine?
"Ma'am, I think there's nothing in it,
It's been broken for a long time!
You'll never get a Coke from that machine!"

As I walked away, my head down,
Angry tears fell on the pavement.
It must be all my fault
That this Coke machine won't work.
It's such a simple process,
Place a quarter, push the button;
It's got to work, I'll get my Coke from this machine!

I said my prayers fervently
Then returned that very evening.
Gaunt from thirst I stood there
Staring at the Coke machine.
Then suddenly around me,
All the Coke machines were calling:
"Try us, we'll give you Coke that he can't give.

We are full and he is empty,
Been that way for quite a long time.
You'd have saved yourself a headache
If you'd come to us before.
He's got trouble on the inside,
'Less he fix it he can't do much,
'Cause a Coke machine can't give what it ain't got."


## GROWTH THROUGH CRISIS

I've been chilled and frozen over the years
By injuries, losses, deprivations and fears.
God's thawed me out from these negative ices
By allowing a major emotional crisis.

One whom I banked on to deliver my joy
Has defrauded me and my trust destroyed.
In the heat of the pain I could not stay frozen,
It was "die or deal" so to deal I have chosen.

I have felt so much anger, sadness and pain!
But I am now dealing, turning losses to gain.
Finding health through forgiveness I'm becoming more free,
I'm deriving much wealth from adversity.

I've been learning how life's big earthquakes can trigger
New courage and growth which like a great river,
Ever widening and deepening as it runs its course,
Exudes greater majesty than at its source. 1993

## FANTASY

I want to be loved by someone
With purpose and passion for life;
A man not double-minded
But constant in his commitment,
Securely embracing all I am
Without a need to belittle me;
A man who will nurture my garden,
Not choke its growth with weeds;
Who will water me lavishly,
Then revel in my blooming;
A man with a dream
Which, merged with mine,
Brings to life a new dimension
We could not separately know.
Then when our dreams are spent,
And time has corroded beauty,
When winter's icy finger beckons me,
And strength's last fading petal softly falls,
He will still be there. 1993

## A NOBLER QUEST

Your unyielding demonstration
Of unrelenting minimization
Has exposed the stark reality
I've shunned but now must see.
You have made clear
There are people held more dear
Than the one who labors to maintain
Your household and your kids sustain.
Thanks for showing to me plainly
That for your love I labored vainly.

So now a nobler quest I make,
Not for your love but for God's sake,
And for the jewels entrusted to my care,
I'll labor on amid the slights and sneers.
There are other dreams for which I have to live,
More promising than what you had to give,
Aspirations far worthier of my effort
Than the cheap substitute for love you offered. 1994


## FORWARD IN FAITH

Lost in a fog of pain and fear,
Not knowing which way I should steer,
I felt shipwrecked and all alone,
Afraid that You too, Lord, had gone.
Winds of rejection stung my spirit,
Waves of defeat rolled right into it,
Battered about by the billows high,
I thought that I would surely die.

Despair clutched at my very brain,
The years, flashed before me, seemed in vain.
Unrelenting tears my garments drenched,
Undiluted sorrows my spirit wrenched.
But You carried me when I didn't know;
How could I see You? I was hurting so!
Yet You lifted me, now new strength You give.
You have eased my pain, made me want to live.

People come and go, but I know You won't,
People let us down, but I know You don't.
I didn't think the pain would ever leave,
That someday its intensity would recede.

This new strength in me, I know where it's from.
Now I want to live till You call me home.
So forward in faith to the upward climb,
I will not turn back, I've made up my mind.

I may stumble on through some valleys dark,
But You'll keep my feet on the proper path
Till you bring me safe to the mountain top,
Where I may at last understand my lot.
So I say, Oh Lord, mold me as You choose,
Make me into a vessel that You can use,
And like Job I say, though You slay, I'll trust.
I'll go on in faith since go on I must.


## LOST VALENTINE

I once had a valentine,
My love for him was genuine;
I pledged to him all of my heart
Sincerely from the very start.

When I committed to be his wife,
My sacred vow was meant for life.
Twelve painful years have passed along
And now my valentine is gone.

I know in this world there are men
Who do not value a rare gem.
They'll step on it, kick it around,
Then leave it laying on the ground.

They'll treat it like some common stone,
Then lunge for an old dried up bone.
I'll never understand such men;
My valentine was one of them.

I once had a valentine
Whose love I thought was genuine.
I trusted in him through and through,
Something a girl should never do.

He plundered the treasures of my soul
As pirates did in days of old,
Then caring naught for what he left,
Like pirate, sought another deck.

My valentine is gone for good;
I can't believe he really could.
I've almost gone mad trying to find
A reason for his great decline.

Why did he leave the upright path,
Breaking and splintering my heart?
Why the self-centeredness displayed?
Why the destructive choices made?

I believe he lost his way,
As all of us are prone to stray
From the path of righteousness
And of our lives make a great mess.

But God is searching for him too
With greater grief and love more true;
He'll find him, put him back on track,
My valentine God will bring back.

I saw his pain, I tried to help,
But in helping was not true to self.
I tried to please but nothing worked,
Rejection in the shadows lurked.

Yet there were times we seemed to meet
In intimacy deep and sweet.
My valentine was sometimes kind,
It seemed his love was genuine.

There was a time I lauded him
As most compassionate of men.
He seemed upright and honest too
In all that he would say and do.

Some tender moments I recall,
When he embraced me and love was all
I felt exuding from him to me.
Were such moments then mere fantasy?

I wish my valentine could know
The love for him that in me flows.
My children daily ask me, "When
Is Daddy coming home again?"

I answer them, "I do not know,
But we'll keep praying till he shows."
The Lord gave wisdom to my son,
He said, "You need more patience, Mom."

A stranger sometimes rings my bell,
But who it is I cannot tell.
He seems familiar, but I'm wrong.
My valentine has been long gone! 1994

# PART 6. JOY IN RECOVERY

## SINK OR SWIM

Those ominous dreams were now fulfilled. Standing without a mate on the deck of a sinking ship, I stared in dismay at the two small children left in my charge. Waves of rejection buffeted the vessel, filling my heart with despair. Pressures of single parenting, financial instability, and fear of the future were pressing in like specters from a bad dream. Invasion of my privacy via the legal system loomed large on the horizon. Would I be compelled to stop homeschooling before I was ready? How long could I stay afloat?

Scared of going under, I reached for a life jacket and began natural progesterone treatment for severe PMS. The transformative results were noticed even by the children. Foolishly I let my guard down (as I was prone to do when he was "nice"), sharing my elation with their father on one of his visits. A drastic reduction in the support check short-circuited that effort. Struggling to keep my head above water, I reached out to a counselor and began taking an antidepressant.

After any hope of reconciliation was shattered by the arrival of divorce papers, I helped the children put on their life jackets, and we three went to family therapy. Although Agalia freely verbalized her fears, she was having sleep problems. Avizi, whether from onset of puberty or pent-up feelings about the family breakdown, or both, was exhibiting out-of-control behavior. They were complaining that we didn't have fun anymore. Their demand for my attention was insatiable, but I was only one parent doing the job meant for two. Counseling helped them understand their value and learn to express their emotions in a healthy way.

Avizi eventually acknowledged his resentment at having more chores than his sister. I understood. We were all angry. The captain had jumped ship. The remaining crew had to assume extra duties to stay afloat. It was natural for me to delegate more responsibilities to the older child. I promised to make some adjustments. We all had fun

113

punching out our frustrations on a dummy in a corner of the therapist's playroom.

My spouse chose to break our vows after 11 years. The journey had taken a sharp detour. The future was uncertain. The choice was obvious, sink or swim. I am recording my vows for posterity. Delusional or not, this is where my heart was in 1980:

"Before God our Father, our families, and friends here present, as the special man that you are, I pledge to you my love and loyalty. I promise to cherish, honor and serve you in ways that will ensure your personal growth and happiness. Joy and prosperity I will share with you. In want, defeat and struggle, I will stand with you. In health and sickness I will care for you, until death takes us one from the other. These vows I make to you, not in my own inadequate strength, but by the power of the loving Lord Jesus who Himself charged me with the privilege and responsibility of loving you as He loves us."

## *OBITUARY*

In painful memory of a man gone mad,
Son, husband, dad,
Whose unbridled passion violently erupting,
Like hot lava, flowed over innocent hearts,
Blistering hope;
A man shunning Truth, running from Grace,
Turning back on blessings.
He leaves behind:
Three souls laid bare to the glare of betrayal,
Vows violated, dreams deferred,
Deep father wound in boy and girl. 1995

## I BROKE MY HEART

If I sustained a broken leg,
Would you order me out of bed?
Would you label me a wimp
If I tried to walk but limped?
If from a fall I broke my back,
Would you make me carry your sack?
Or would you bring me "Meals on Wheels,"
Be my companion while I heal?
Now alas, I broke my heart!
It seems that I must mourn apart
From friends that I had thought would care.
There aren't very many here,
And some have said, "Snap out of it!"
They can't abide a broken spirit.


## GOD SENDS NEW FRIENDS

Nursing a broken heart and suffering deep emotional insecurity, I felt shunned by some I thought were friends. They would have been perfectly fine if I could have hidden my pain. I couldn't, so they disappeared. Others were playing the blame game without knowing the facts. Mere acquaintances assumed the right to pass judgement on matters that were none of their business.

I lived with the stigma of divorce. People generally seem more responsive to the pain caused by death or illness than they are to the pain of divorce. The church we were attending never reached out to us beyond requests for the pastor's love offering. The usual Saturday evening call to ask if the children would be in Sunday school didn't come anymore. A couple we considered friends had sometimes driven us to church when my spouse went out of town. I was bewildered when they refused us rides after the separation.

Roslyn was the only friend who showed up on the day my husband left. She brought dinner for the children and me and stayed until he walked out the door, possibly preventing another emotional altercation. When Pamela's husband died, she was surrounded by friends and supporters all evening. My grief was as intense as hers. Why was the response so different? Pamela found closure in burying her loved one; while grieving, she could move on with her life. My *loved one,* even after our marriage was dead, continued complicating my life and intensifying my suffering.

A week after the separation, Lisa joined our homeschool group. She invited us to her church, offering to pick us up the following Sunday. For the next year, she and her husband gave us rides to church each week, stopping only when their son was about to be born. Nichole stepped in as a new friend and helper, and we discovered that our daughters shared the same birthday. They are still best friends 25 years later. Nichole and I have also maintained an enduring friendship. Ellen, the church bus driver for many years, became my friend and later, my caregiver.

Grateful as I am for all who supported me, I realize that my strength comes not just from people support, but from God, the ultimate Provider. When my fleeing spouse slammed one door in my face, God opened another to let in those who would truly care. The divorce helped weed out superficial friends, making room for genuine and lasting relationships.

## A LIGHTHOUSE IN OUR STORM

We came broken, rejected, in pain and despair,
Some of us wondering if God was still there.
Betrayal and failure was the banner we bore,
Our hearts were shattered, bleeding and sore.

But God, in His grace, had gone on before us,
Clearing a path, opening doors for us.
He had prepared to help pick up the pieces,
To wrap up the wounds and put balm on the bruises.

You're one of those people He's specially gifted
With a caring heart which so many has lifted.
You're creative, versatile, blessed with a sharp mind,
Yet friendly, transparent, humble and kind.

We have cried to you, feeling unloved and neglected,
Yet never felt condemned nor rejected.
You've taught us how to best profit from pain,
How to grieve our losses and live again.

We didn't agree with all that you said,
But you mostly hit the nail on the head.
And there are some occasions we remember
When you missed the nail and hit your finger.

You are going because it is in God's plan,
Your life and future are secure in His hands.
The seeds you have sown will reap plentiful harvest,
As the lives you have rescued will in turn others bless.

Dedicated to Pastor Tom, who supported me through divorce recovery.

## *YOUR LIFE HAS TOUCHED MINE*

I was going mad inside my head,
Spending sleepless nights upon my bed.
My reality was all askew.
Which way was up I wished I knew.
Then I went to see one preacher man
And left crazier than I began.

I tried again, looked for another,
Hoping he'd do better than the other,
Hoping someone would hear me out,

Hoping I wouldn't have to shout
My protests to the wind again,
That someone would my truth defend.

Who could imagine my consternation
When accounts of betrayal and violation
Were scrutinized and simplified,
Misinterpreted and minimized?
I felt devalued and misunderstood,
Felt evil would triumph over good.

"There are problems, man, don't you understand?
I can't cover them up, I've done that too long.
Big problems, man, they make heartstrings break!"
I just cried and cried, my whole being ached.
He denied the seriousness of things,
Thought a few pat answers would healing bring.

Then hopelessness took root and grew,
Clinging to everything I knew,
Until I met another man
From whose caring new hope sprang.
A quiet man he was, not ostentatious,
A humble man and very gracious.

He let me express my pain and grief,
His validation brought great relief.
He confirmed for me the worst fears I had,
Acknowledged the problem was very bad.
And ah, my sanity slowly returned,
As my concerns were no longer spurned.

On days when I hurt and would the walls climb,
You were on the other end of the line.
You counseled, encouraged, admonished, directed,
Prayed earnestly for and always supported

My children and me through many a trial,
Brought me back to reality from denial.

You're a wise and godly man, I know
And you will bless others wherever you go.
You have a big heart and you've shared it with me,
In you God's love and compassion I see.
Your life has touched mine in a powerful way,
Far more than these words can ever say.

Dedicated to Pastor Ron Butler, 1933-2015

## YOU ARE LIKE THE SUNSHINE

You have been so good to us
That we can scarcely find
Words to express the gratitude
That's in our hearts and minds.
You are like the sunshine
On a cloudy day,
Your cheerfulness and kindness
Help drive the gloom away.
It's so very comforting
Knowing that you are there,
Having such friends to lean on
When burdened with life's cares.
May God bless you and reward you
For the thoughtful things you do.
The world would sure be better
If filled with people just like you. 1995

Dedicated to Rosie & Dave
Thanks for sending my kids to summer camp.

## *JOY IN THE MORNING*

My heart has been trampled and broken,
Pain in my soul runs deep,
For the man I once trusted to love me
His commitment has failed to keep.
He has ransacked my innermost being,
Smeared graffiti all over the wall,
He has blasted dreams I once cherished,
Ripped treasures from memory's hall.

Another, far greater than he is,
Has picked me up off the floor.
He has put His arms gently around me,
Saying, "Joy, for you, there is more!
Dreams that are greater than those gone
I will conceive in your heart.
Hold on, trust Me, for I'll heal you
And give you a brand new start.

Stay focused on Me, your Sustainer,
For My love is true to the end.
I will comfort, restore and affirm you,
Till with strength you again can stand.
The stories you'll tell when I've healed you
Will draw many people to Me,
For those who are broken and hurting
Will in you, My Omnipotence see.

Only I can give beauty for ashes
Or unravel tangled strands,
Bring harmony out of discord,
Or cause the mourner to dance.
Only I can bring joy in the morning,
After nights of weeping and pain.
Only I can again make the sun shine,
After a long season of rain. 1995

"…Weeping may remain for a night, but rejoicing comes in the morning." Psalm 30:5b

## *RECLAMATION*

You're there for me, I see it every day,
You're not two-faced about the things You say,
You know just what You want, You're not confused,
You shower me with love and not abuse.
Even when I'm weak, You hang around,
And if I fall, You lift me off the ground.
Although my rebel heart is prone to stray,
You do remember that I am but clay.

When I come back to You, my head held low,
You never chide or scold, "I told you so!"
But wrap me in Your mercy as You say:
"I'm glad you're back, I hope you're home to stay.
I've been waiting here so long to see you come
And feel the tender embrace of My arms.
It's Me you need, I'm genuine through and through,
I'll meet your needs, I'll not abandon you.

I value you far more than any can
And I do not deceive, I Am not man.
In My arms you needn't cringe, so do be real!
Whatever makes your heart hurt I will heal.
So come, reclaim the territory lost to pain.
I'll make your losses all turn into gain.
Your woundedness I'll use to help heal others,
To lift a fallen sister or a brother.

Like Me, you will become a wounded healer,
And the purpose of your lot will be much clearer,
As through you My compassion I will send,
And lives touched by your own begin to mend."
With heartfelt gratitude I now reclaim
Everything that's mine in Jesus' name.
In the comfort of Your love I now will rest,
And in Your strength I'll stand, whatever the test! 1995


"…Go and enjoy choice food and sweet drinks…Do not grieve, for the joy of the Lord is your strength." Nehemiah 8:10


## MY ONE TRUE LOVE

Patiently You've waited all this time,
Your tender eyes embracing me,
Wondering when I would the truth receive.
Thank You for Your pure unselfish love
That gives me freedom to be who I am.
You encourage me to show my giftedness
Without the scalding tones of minimization,
Always delighting in my success.
Remove the fear that makes me doubt
The deep dimensions of Your love for me.
Put to rout with the breath of Your mouth
Those who would assail me.
Hold me firmly in Your strong embrace
Till my heart no longer wanders,
Lured by glitter of fool's gold
Or empty packages proffered by the world.
Then my soul at last will find repose,
Its confidence and security in You. 1995

"How priceless is your unfailing love!" Psalm 36:7

# CELEBRATING A COVENANT

When rheumatoid arthritis began to lay siege against Mama's body, little did we know what a long, painful battle it would be. As the doctors launched their chemical counterattack, her body reacted. Drugs were added to drugs until she succumbed to diabetes and lupus. As the arthritis advanced, Mama's ability to function slowly diminished.

Mama came to help when Avizi was born. She was on her feet bustling around the house. When Agalia was almost two, Daddy and Mama spent Christmas with us. She was walking with a cane and had to rest frequently, but I couldn't keep her out of the kitchen. While we were in Boston following the separation, Mama alternated between a cane and a walker and did much of her cooking sitting down. Near the end of our stay, Mama was admitted to the hospital with pneumonia. Determined to return home before we left, she did just that. In the ensuing months, her body continued to weaken. She was in and out of the hospital.

"It will be very hard for you," the doctor told Daddy, delivering the shocking diagnosis. Mama had Alzheimer's disease. Ivy and Claudius had been married for almost 50 years. Daddy had anticipated celebrating their golden anniversary. He now realized that even if Mama lived, she probably wouldn't be able to appreciate the event or even attend. Wanting to honor his queen in a big way one last time, Daddy made a decision.

In December 1995, Avizi, Agalia and I arrived at the homestead in Boston to spend Christmas and celebrate our parents' 48th wedding anniversary. We suspected it would be our last Christmas with Mama. The preceding six months had been difficult. Daddy had reserved a venue for the function, but had to cancel. Phone calls were made to inform guests of the change. The church hall was crowded, but it didn't dampen the spirit of celebration that prevailed on December 31st.

Shocked at the fragile hands that grasped mine, I hugged her gingerly, afraid of breaking her protruding bones. Mama, size 16 in her prime, had shrunk to size eight. With assistance and great effort, she got out of bed, shuffled with her walker to the kitchen, and sat with us as we ate breakfast. In order to keep her spirits up, Daddy had told her that everybody was coming.

Seeming very happy, she suddenly asked, "So when is Joy coming?" It took me off guard. Mama didn't know who I was. The reality was not an easy one to handle. The realization that I was losing my mother sunk in. A part of me went numb.

As siblings arrived with their offspring, the hullabaloo increased. Mama was sitting on the sofa. She seemed to be in another world. Suddenly, she waved her hand. My nephews were playing Nintendo and Faith had inadvertently blocked her view. We all chortled in surprise.

Agalia, just nine years old, commented, "Grandma seems to be brighter since we arrived." All the noise and excitement must have been stimulating. Daddy was an attentive caregiver, but he couldn't meet all her needs. Being diabetic, he had his own set of health issues.

Daddy was delighted to have us all at home. In the midst of the merriment, he added to the din, playing the piano and singing his favorite songs. He paused intermittently to respond to the grandkids' requests for Mama's Ensure pudding. When the noise became too much, Grandpa tried in vain to quiet the kids. Then remembering, "If you can't beat them, join them," he marched up and down the hallway, proclaiming, "Follow your leader!" The grandchildren fell in line behind Grandpa, their giggles effervescing into uproarious laughter. What a riot! We caught the memory on video.

The big day came. Mama was attractively adorned in a bright pink dress that complemented her fair complexion, accessorized with white hat and gloves. Too feeble to walk down the stairs, she was transported in Danny's arms. It was an emotional moment for Danny, as he recalled all the times Mama had carried him physically, emotionally and spiritually.

Like the queen that she was, Ivy waved to the audience as Danny carried her to her seat up front next to Daddy. I was awed by the significance of the moment. We were celebrating the 48-year covenant of two people who were, I am proud to say, my parents. It was important for my children to know an example of enduring commitment.

To the surprise and delight of my parents, children and grandchildren participated in a program of floral and oral tributes, music and poetry. Of my three brothers and three sisters, two were missing. Paul was not well; he rehearsed with us but was a no-show for the event. Grace, her husband and three children resided in Jamaica. Thanks to modern technology, we broadcast her family's tributes to Mama and Daddy via speakerphone.

Daniel (D2) was the only other missing grandchild. His father, Daniel (D1), was the M.C. for the evening; Patrick (aka Taqwa) was his co-host. They entertained the audience with their comical repartee. My nephew, Jamal, owned a keyboard with a prerecorded reggae tune— "I Shot the Sheriff." A few days before the celebration, Jamal and I borrowed the tune and composed lyrics that paid homage to his grandparents.

"I love my Grandpa,
And I also love my Grandma too, oh yeah!
I love them so!
How much? You'll never know!
For dey always care for me
Even when I was baby."

Cheers erupted, as children and grandchildren swayed and clapped to the rhythm of the beat, singing with gusto. Each grandchild (Avizi, Agalia, Jamal, Jeremy, Jonathan, Joanna and Jarrick) sang solo, passing the mike to each other. My siblings (Carol, Danny, Patrick, Faith) and I exchanged "Grandpa" and "Grandma" with "Me Fada" and "Me Mada." The audience chanted with enthusiasm when Faith invited them to sing to Mas Claudie and Miss Ivy.

Patrick lauded Daddy for being the "Psalm 1 Man," a one-woman man, and a fitting role model. The place was ablaze with laughter when he shared his version of why my parents chose our names.

"Joy, you see, was first and decided to come feet first. She gave Mama a hard time and it was a joy when that ordeal ended, so she called the baby Joy. She needed grace to deal with Joy, so the second baby was named Grace. After Carol, came Paul, Daniel and myself; to deal with us three, God knows, she had to have Faith." Mama was smiling and clapping. I was actually named when my mom's cousin heard of my arrival and declared, "Oh what a joy! Let's call her Joy!"

Agalia read Psalm 23, Mama's favorite, and Jamal read Psalm 8, Daddy's favorite. Carol and I each sang solos, while Faith offered a fitting oral tribute, honoring Claudius and Ivy for their faithful commitment to God, to each other, and to their offspring. Avizi gave flowers to his grandparents on behalf of the grandchildren. An elder of the church presented an engraved plaque to the couple, commemorating their 27 years of faithful service.

Daddy had not anticipated "such a wonderful evening." He was profuse in his thanks to everyone for their overwhelming show of friendship and encouragement. He took us on a journey back to the days of his courtship. Spellbound, the crowd hung on every word, their feedback goading him on.

After retiring downstairs for an elegantly catered dinner, we enjoyed recalling amusing incidents from our childhood and tattling on each other. Much of this was done in our Jamaican *patwa*, making it even more comical, since the audience was mostly of Caribbean descent. Several of us shared poems written in honor of Ivy, our Poet-in-Chief.

As the evening ended, Mama surprised us by giving a closing speech in her usual poetic style. She recognized that her earthly sojourn was coming to a close, though she wasn't sure when. What she was sure of was that "we will all meet again, and no one will have the authority to separate us." Ivy reminded us that she was not looking for the undertaker, but for the "Upper-taker." One day she would go, "not in a plane that can crash, or in a limo that can get a flat, or in a bus that has to stop." She would be flying "straight through to Glory!" Mama thanked everyone from the "smallest child to the grey head," as she ran her fingers through Daddy's salt & pepper hair. It was her last public speech, recorded for posterity.

After Daddy's closing remarks and a prayer, the festivities ended with resounding applause.

Daddy's sweetness of spirit and patient care of Mama during her long illness is worthy of praise. Caring for Mama at home was a demanding task, but Daddy never complained. She was his queen and he did not want her to suffer indignities so often rampant in nursing homes. Some men don't stick around for their children to grow up, much less for their wives to grow old. My siblings and I were fortunate to have parents who remained faithful to each other for so many years. I failed to procure that blessing for my children— a sad regret indeed!

Ivy and Claudius lived exemplary lives, though not without conflict, disappointment or failure. They honored their covenant to God and to each other, understanding that, what mattered was not the smoothness of the road, but that two agreed to travel together to the end.


## TRIBUTE TO OUR FATHER

This is a tribute to Claud,
A man who deserves great applaud,
A man who worked hard day and night.
With godly wisdom and insight,
Three sons he did raise right,
Although at times the task was quite a fight.

Each son was quite unique, each had his own mystique.
The three at times were hard to understand.
There was Patrick, the quiet ponderer;
Paul, the happy wanderer;
And Danny, who was from birth a lady's man.
Pat pondered things profound, Paul traveled all around,
While Dan charmed all the pretty girls in town.
They almost drove Claud crazy; Claud, who was never lazy,
Earned every grey hair in his glorious crown,

So this tribute we must pay.
To Claud, our dad, we say,
From your three pains in the neck,
"Happy Father's Day!"—Taqwa The Edutainer (Patrick) ©1991


## *MOTHER DEAR*

Earth never had a gem so rare,
So precious as my mother dear,
Her sacrifices made for me
Are more than eye will ever see.

In thick and thin she's by my side,
I never can my sorrows hide.
In spite of failure on my part,
She always shows a loving heart.

I used to think she nagged too much,
But now I know why all the fuss.
All her desires are for me
That I'll a perfect woman be.

When I might have gone astray,
She did not forget to pray.
No other one can love me more
Nor like her all my faults endure.

Lord, bless my mother with the thought
That I'll not turn from what she's taught,
But will, through Thine own strength divine,
As a beacon in this dark world shine. 1970

## *ASPIRATIONS*

If you can trust yourself when others doubt you
And conquer fears that limit what you dare;
If you can freely give to those around you
The gifts and talents that are yours to share;
If you can live, not for your pleasure only,
But gladly lend your gentleness and grace
To warm the hearts of people who are lonely
And help to make the world a better place;
If you can balance dreams with practicality,
Can deal in facts yet never lose ideals;
If you can face the harshness of reality
And find the truth that prejudice conceals;
If you can be courageous when defeated
And humble in the face of victory;
And give your best until a task's completed,
However difficult that task may be;
If you can temper knowledge with understanding
And seek to gently guide, not to control,
Then neither be too lax nor too demanding,
But understand the worth of every soul;
If you can look beyond the faults of others
To see their need for mercy and for grace;
If you can then forgive and not be bothered
To seek your "pound of flesh," help them save face,
A noble soul you'll be, a breath from Heaven,
An emissary from God's throne of grace,
A light to some, for others hope rekindled,
A life that will not have been lived in vain.

Dedicated to Ivy Lucilda Walker, Oct. 10, 1917-Oct. 31, 1996

*Joy Walker*

## THE BIRDS GIVE THANKS

One evening in the month of May,
As the sun was sinking slowly
Behind the clustered trees,
Making way for the moon and stars
To master the night as God ordained,
The birds flew about and seemed to say,
"Thank God for the sun that ruled the day,
The God who gave us food today
And springs of water on our way.
He teaches us our young to feed
Though nestled helpless in a tree."
The birdies chirp, the birds spread out
Their small protective wings
And seemed to say, "Great things
The Lord has done for us!" 1966

(Written by Mama and Joy)


## GOD WILL WORK IT ALL OUT

Sometimes changes come into our lives
That we neither want nor welcome.
We may pout or shake our fists at God
Or kick up our heels in a tantrum.
No matter who or what is to blame
For bringing the change about,
We must be convinced in our hearts at last
That God will work it all out.

We must believe that He's in control,
That His wisdom is unlimited,
Yet He never promised a bed of ease
Or that dreams would go un-aborted.

So no matter the turn or twist in the road
That seems to throw us off course,
We must be convinced in our hearts at last
That God will work it all out.

Even when our present pain and *dis-ease*
Results from our own rebellion,
And in guilt we try to run from God
Or fix things by our own understanding,
Even then, if we turn with penitent heart
To embrace His truth and grace,
We must be convinced in our hearts at last
That God will work it all out.

Yes, changes will come into our lives
We can neither avert nor hinder.
We must grieve the losses those changes bring,
Acknowledge the feelings they kindle.
But don't let them rattle your faith in the Lord
For through all, He remains changeless,
And be convinced in your heart at last
That for good, God will work it all out.


## WHEN DADDY LEFT
(Seen through the eyes of my daughter)

When Daddy left he didn't say, but I know why.
I sometimes listened, ear to wall, heard Mama cry.
I wished that Dad would love her more,
But he just walked right out the door.

He didn't leave just Mama here, or don't I count?
I feel so sad inside my heart I want to shout,
"Don't you even care about my pain?"
But Dad's already married again.

Now Daddy has another home and I know why.
I guess I wasn't good enough but I sure tried.
My mama says it isn't true,
That grown-ups sometimes mess up too.

Dad says we live in luxury and have too much.
I think he thinks that Mama has a lot of stuff.
I tried to tell him all we need,
But he just shrugged and called it greed.

Daddy's new marriage didn't work, he must be blue.
But why he keeps on messing up, I have no clue.
I'll have to talk to God again,
I am confused, it makes no sense.

Sometimes I feel so very sad but don't know why.
I guess I really miss my dad but I can't cry.
I'll ask God to let Daddy know
I love him and I need him so! 1996

## A GARDENER'S PRAYER

Rare flower buds You've given me
To nurture and to cultivate.
I water them with love and prayers
And hedge them in with discipline.
May I not too busy be
Nor fail their loveliness to see,
And may I linger to inhale
The fragrance of their blooming.

Fortify me through the years
As I tend them with patient care.
May every petal stay in place
Regardless of the storms that come.

May neither blight nor wind nor heat
Cause them to wither at my feet,
And may they, rooted in Your grace,
Draw life and sustenance from the sun.

As the gardener, may I enjoy
The harvest of my life's long toil,
Rare flowers that are in full bloom,
Examples of Your sovereignty,
The stunning beauty of lives well-lived,
Undaunted by adversity.

## HEARTBREAK

The pain's diminished but not gone,
Like low-grade fever it lingers on,
Often threatening ominously
To overtake and swallow me.

Sometimes I stare as if in a trance
While snapshots of life before me dance,
Then, unsolicited, tears copious flow
At memory of betrayal's blow.

Sometimes I relinquish a thousand sighs
From tension building up inside.
Sometimes the pain without warning comes
Like a jagged knife that's roughly plunged.

Sometimes a dull and endless ache
Like heartburn, keeps me wide awake.
Sometimes I trudge on step by step
From sheer habit and not with zest.

Sometimes stiff jaw and upper lip
Is how I manage to exist,
And as life moves on in ebbs and flows,
So the pain, it comes and goes.

"My grace is sufficient for you, for my power is made perfect in weakness." 2 Corinthians 12:9

# PART 7. CONFOUNDING CONUNDRUM

## *THE PLEDGE OF A FRIEND*

I need a heart that's open to my gaze,
A heart not filled with devious ways,
To whom I can say, "Here is who I am,
I'll show you all of me, love me if you can."

I need earnest eyes that with hopefulness shine,
Full of compassion, keenly looking into mine,
Peering past the flimsy camouflage of a painted smile
To discover my broken spirit, dreams that have almost died.

I need eager ears to listen as again and again
In emotional catharsis I pour out my pain.
I need strong arms that will steady my step
As I sway 'neath the load life has heaped on my breast.

I need genuine connection with someone who cares,
Who will laugh and cry with me and always be there,
Who won't try to say when my grieving should end.
What I need, I believe, is the pledge of a friend.

"A friend loves at all times, and a brother is born for adversity."
Proverbs 17:17


## *DEEDLESS WORDS*

I will not live for deedless words
Brushed from your table like crumbs for dogs,
Flung out to momentarily save face,
Then quickly nullified by deprecating actions;

135

Words for the mindless fool who rushes to embrace
A gaudy, empty bauble.
I will not live life cheaply,
Banking principle on a mirage
Created by your hollow platitudes
To charm the unsuspecting;
Promises that promenade like prize horses
Then stumble under scrutiny.


## THE WOMEN AND THE MEN

There is trouble in the air and it is serious.
It's the women and the men and they are furious.
Whatever can we do, does anybody have a clue?
The heat is so intense, I am delirious.

To say "boys will be boys," that isn't fair to us.
They treat us just like toys, that's what they do to us.
Today they'll play with one and discard her when they're done,
Then tomorrow they will find some more at "*Toys for Us.*"

All the women should be friends, it's really up to us.
If they had no place to go, they'd give the matter up.
We must stop this gross abuse, don't let men our bodies use,
Then this disrespect would stop and they would honor us.


## I DON'T KNOW WHY

I know you're hurting and I am too,
But there's room in my heart to care for you.
You may push away the love I share,
But you can't intercept my prayer.

You've shown me the pain in your aching soul
And I wish that pain I could control.
I'd take it away, that's what I'd do,
But it seems that I heighten the pain in you.

I just don't know why life is this way,
Why living and loving make us pay
Such a great price in grief and fear,
Why the pathway so often seems unclear.

Yet I'm committed to love and life
Even with its cares and pain and strife,
For I'd rather be a heart that's risking still
Than a heart alive, yet atrophied. 1995


## *ANNIVERSARY OF A FRIENDSHIP*

We've been friends long enough to have peered past
The pleasing camouflage of best foot forward,
To see the imperfections of each other's person.
We have felt the heat from rough edges in motion,
Tasted the bitter sweetness of hearts exposed to scrutiny,
And tripped in the pothole of enmeshed emotions.
Daunted by the crippling fear of intimacy,
We've measured the limits of our friendship.
Let's adjust our hope for this relationship,
Accepting what it is and what it's not.

# MANHOLE

I was trudging along in the heat of the day when I came to an intersection. Pondering which way to go, I noticed that one direction led down a cozy, shady lane, where the branches of the trees intertwined, providing comforting protection from the ravaging sun. I sauntered down this pleasant path, filling my nostrils with the refreshing scent of greenery. Meandering along, enchanted by the sunbeams playfully dancing through the leaves, I missed the hole.

Horrified, I looked up and saw it was a long way to the top. After much effort, I pulled myself out and limped on. Despite the pain, I really enjoyed walking down this road. Next time I would be more careful to avoid the hole.

Next time came and again, entranced by my alluring surroundings, I missed the hole and fell in. Managing to grab the sides, I avoided hitting bottom. I was angry with myself for being so careless! At first, I had assumed the lane was safe. Enthralled by its ambiance, I didn't bother to check for signs of danger. There was now no excuse. I needed to be more careful. Perhaps I was in denial, because I continued traveling that road, allowing myself to be charmed into negating the danger.

Finally, I became tired of the pain, of the wounds I was nursing. Couldn't I go another way? As cozy as it seemed, this path was not safe. The hole would always be there. It was time to change course. But what was my hesitation? Was it the protection from the heat that this road afforded? That was a reasonable consideration. What about the repeated pain of falling? Was it worth a few moments of pleasure? I considered other options and made my decision.

Now I walk "the road less traveled," where the light is bright and the heat intense, but there are no potholes, no possibility of falling. Oh, by the way, I almost forgot to mention the man whose magnetism kept pulling me toward the hole. It took all the strength in me to escape his clutches. Though he tried to impede my escape, I couldn't entirely blame him. The problem was mine to solve and I did. The choice I made was prudent—no more *manholes* for me!

## ON THE REBOUND

The heat was hot upon my head,
Life's journey I had come to dread,
Abandoned and in deepest pain
I thought his coming was my gain.

With flowery words and gifts he came,
I knew not that his heart was lame,
I was in medicated stupor,
He then seemed like such a trooper.

I trusted, opened up my heart,
Believed him from the very start,
The care he showed I needed, sure!
Then I found out he needed more.

The things I once received from him
Have question marks all over them.
I've learned his gifts have strings attached
So now, those strings I'll have to cut.

The boundaries are back in place,
I'd rather be alone and safe,
I'll not entertain unhealthy men,
Not now and I hope never again! 1996


## I BELIEVE IN ME

The roller coaster of your double-talking
Kept me reeling with uncertainty.
Now I'm down, feet firmly on the ground.
My heart's again believing in only what is real.
Things you said I'm sorting through, tossing what's untrue.
The positive I'll cherish, but your negativity leaves with you.

## *PEOPLE-PLEASER NO MORE!*

I heard somewhere a message that I wasn't good enough.
I've met in life some people to whom I couldn't give enough.
I tried so hard to please them that I was false to self.
I believed if I could give enough I'd find love for myself.

I hadn't heard the message that I must love me first.
I believed that other people would give me my self-worth.
I believed that if I pleased them, I would find significance,
But my efforts were unfruitful though I did this deadly dance.

I've internalized the message that was sent from God above.
He established my significance when He gave to me His love,
A love so unconditional, accepting me as I am,
A love so inspirational, showing me who I can become.

I strive today to please Him in right relationship
With Him, myself and others in gratitude for His gift.
I confront the sin in others as well as in myself
And put boundaries on evil, so I can be true to self.

## SELF-ACCEPTANCE

Many of us, driven by an overwhelming need for approval, harbor a negative self-image and spend our lives trying to be like somebody else or vainly trying to please others. We fail to recognize our value in God's eyes. Everything God creates has a special function and place in His plan. Everything God creates is good. Of course we must acknowledge that God's good creation has been warped by sin. This is why Jesus had to come, in order to redeem and restore what has been broken. When we seek and find God, we also will find fulfillment in the purpose for which we were made.

God gave me a disability for His own purposes. I can spend my days grumbling about it, or I can glorify God by blossoming in my designated sphere. When I contend with God regarding my genetic endowment, social and parental heritage, or innate abilities, I fail to appreciate that these are all divine gifts. Discontentment creates a barrier in my relationship with the Giver who desires and deserves my gratitude.

Negative self-criticism never leads to joy. Fulfillment begins at the cross of Jesus Christ. God's love for us is demonstrated in the sacrifice of His Son. When we surrender to that love, then we can truly acknowledge the value He has put on our souls and learn to love ourselves. God calls those who respond to His love "precious and honored" (Isaiah 43:4).

We tend to focus only on our physical well-being, but God places greater value on our spiritual welfare. He wants to build His character into us. Joni Erickson Tada puts it this way: "God is the Master Artist and we are His painting; His model is Jesus Christ, whose very image God wants to paint into our lives. Sometimes a crude, dark line appears in the picture which makes us think He doesn't know what He's doing. Confident of our own ability, we grab the brush from the Artist's hand, jump off the easel and proceed to paint our own picture. Who ever heard of a painting painting a painting?" Joni, a quadriplegic and visual artist, further states that the dark lines which at first seemed like a terrible mistake would have ultimately enhanced the picture. In our impatience and mistrust of the Master Artist's ability, we mess up what could have been a beautiful picture.

God created me with a special purpose in mind and is still perfecting me. I am not what I used to be, nor yet all I will become. I cannot fulfill your purpose; nor can you fulfill mine. We are each distinctly gifted by God and strategically positioned in His plan. I will abandon the habit of negative self-criticism and trust the Master Designer's ability and promise to make all things beautiful in His time. I will cease striving to please others and embrace the person God created me to be.

"For we are God's workmanship, created in Christ Jesus to do good works, which God prepared in advance for us to do." Ephesians 2:10

# PART 8. SISTER TWISTER

## *STILL I LIVE*

If all my tears shed in this life
Were gathered in one flow,
I'd perish in its deluge,
But in His mercy God did not
Allow all grief to strike at once.
If all the pain that pierced my heart
Had at the same time struck,
Suffering would have been brief
With permanent relief.
Yet still I live and still I cry,
Tears mingling with scars hardening
To build resistance for the next attack.
A numb facade at times obscures emotions,
Enabling me to trudge through tedious chores
With occasional eruption of sobs aimed at Heaven,
Queries to the Almighty about the meaning of it all.

"I have loved you with an everlasting love; I have drawn you
with unfailing kindness." Jeremiah 31:3, 4

## HELP IN THE NICK OF TIME

In 1995, while still homeschooling my daughter, I started
attending classes at the Braille Institute. It was a juggling act. On the
days I went to class, I left my daughter with another homeschool
mom and picked her up on the way back. The transportation service
for people with disabilities could be a blight or a blessing. Although
classes ended at three o'clock, one day, the taxi finally reached our
home at 7:30 PM. We were exhausted and stressed out.

Learning Windows 95 was challenging, although I recognized how much the computer would ameliorate the writing process. I was still using an electric typewriter. My goal was to transfer all the poems I had written to the computer, a huge task. A friend helped me format all the poems that I had scribbled or typed over the years. This would make it easier for me to scan each one into the computer.

The members of the writing class (including the instructor) were blind or visually impaired. We were assisted by sighted volunteers. Mac Riley, the instructor, gave positive feedback and encouraged me to keep writing.

Occasionally there were lunchtime concerts where various artists performed. The computer instructor asked me to share the poem "Turn Me Loose." A friend of hers played bongo drums in rhythm with the lilting cadence of my slow rap. As I progressed, the audience became excited. I had struck a chord with the women. They could relate to the sentiments being expressed. I was describing the fight for autonomy and desire for time to indulge my creativity. The sewing instructor was elated.

"Joy, that was fantastic! I wish you could have seen all the women jumping from their chairs. You really were a hit. You should do a live recording."

In the fall of 1996, I was sitting in the student lounge. It was past lunchtime, and I should have been in my computer class. An overwhelming feeling of exhaustion glued me to the chair. A student queried, "Are you okay?" I shook my head as tears flowed freely. He asked, "Would you like me to call someone?" I nodded and soon a staff member was at my side, questioning me with great concern. I agreed to talk to a counselor, who guided me to her office, made me a cup of tea, and then listened.

My mother's declining health had us on an emotional roller coaster for the last year. My ex-spouse was taking me to court a year after the divorce. I was emotionally and physically frazzled. These crises were added to the already formidable demands of being a legally-blind single parent.

"Your plate is full and overflowing. I think you need some help. Have you ever heard of In-House Services? The state provides help for disabled persons with limited income through In-House Supportive Services (IHSS)." I was nervous about bringing a stranger into my home but knew I needed help. The counselor scheduled an appointment with a social worker. I filled out the application and received a list of potential providers.

Clarissa started working for me in October 1996. This was no coincidence. There is a saying that God never gives us more than we can bear. Things went from bad to worse that month. God knew I would not have been able to manage on my own, so He sent Clarissa right in the nick of time.

Not long after, just before a planned weekend getaway, Faith called. The doctor didn't think Mama would last the night. I panicked. Questions swirled through my mind: What should I do? Do I cancel the retreat? Do I wait and see? How much would a ticket cost? What about the children? Mama survived the night. I went to the retreat on pins and needles. The following week, the children and I left for Boston.

If there was ever a time I needed assistance, it was then. Clarissa, a conscientious and empathetic helper, stayed with me for two years before leaving to continue her education.

"I will sing of the Lord's great love forever; with my mouth I will make your faithfulness known through all generations. I will declare that your love stands firm forever..." Psalm 89:1, 2

## THE ONLY MAN WHO CAN

Lord, to You I humbly plead,
I want You to meet my need,
For I've tried the other ways
Which have led my heart astray.

Lord, please mend my broken heart,
To my life, bring a fresh start.
Give me zest and hope for life
Though I'm now a divorced wife.

You're my husband, Lord, it's true,
You're always there when I need You,
You've always showed me that You care,
For I have proof in answered prayer.

When I'm weak, on You I'll lean,
When I'm angry, to You I'll scream.
All my fears You'll understand,
You are the only man who can.

"For your Maker is your husband, the Lord Almighty is his name..." Isaiah 54:5

# END OF HOMESCHOOLING

1996 saw the end of homeschooling and the beginning of public school for my baby girl, who was now ten years old. Avizi had started seventh grade at our church school the previous year. Since I couldn't afford tuition for two, Agalia entered fifth grade at the neighborhood elementary school. Not wanting her to feel that her brother was receiving preferential treatment, we struck a deal. If she earned good grades, I would transfer her after his graduation from eighth grade. She reluctantly agreed and frequently reminded me of my promise.

A nervous little girl grasped my hand as we walked to school on her first day. Returning home, she babbled about the events of the day. A kind student had shown her around and introduced her to some of her friends. The next day a confident, eager girl bounded out the door, urging me to hurry. She was doing just fine.

Agalia's first assignment was to complete a creative writing story. She was motivated and worked diligently. The following day, she came home wilted and distraught. The students had read their stories in class, and the teacher had applauded all except hers.

"Some of the stories weren't even good, Mom, but she said 'excellent' to them." My child was so upset! I reassured her that her story was good; I knew she had tried hard and God knew too. When I related my daughter's distress to the teacher, she, I believe, feigned ignorance.

"I always applaud my students no matter how silly their stories are," she cooed. "I just don't know how that could have happened. I really don't remember that." She promised to talk to Agalia about it but never did. Initially, I had given her the benefit of the doubt, but I felt negative vibes emanating from her to me. On Back-to-School Night, I again felt those vibes as she slithered through her "I always..." and "I never..." statements, endeavoring to impress the parents. Agalia said she told the class on the first day, "I never yell," and kept yelling ever since. She was saying it again to the parents.

"I want the students to be happy. After all, they are only fifth graders. I never want them to cry over homework. If they don't understand something, they can always talk to me the next day and I'll go over it." Agalia shook her head. "Not true!"

I asked the teacher at which reading level she had placed Agalia. She hadn't placed her because, "since she has not been to school before, I have no way of knowing what her reading level was." The previous year, Agalia had tested PHS (post-high school) on the Standard Achievement Test. I wanted her placed at an advanced level to keep her challenged. The test scores had been submitted at registration, but no one had bothered to look at them. Certain negative assumptions had been made when the teacher discovered that my daughter was homeschooled.

Agalia was retested, and the administrator was floored by her extensive vocabulary. My request was subsequently honored, and my child was placed at a reading level commensurate with her ability.

147

# WHEN IT RAINS IT POURS

It was April 12th, 1996. That night, I had a dream. In this dream, I met my ex's new wife for the first time. She seemed formidable, while he sat passively in a corner holding their new baby. From their front porch, as far as I could see, there was water, turbulent water. It was raining heavily. I became very troubled in my spirit and wondered how I would ever cross the water to safety. Would they let me drown? The dream ended.

All next day I cried but wasn't sure why. A friend reminded me it was April 13th, five years to the day since the separation. Later that day Agalia came home very upset. Her daddy's new wife had, allegedly, launched a verbal tirade against her and then smiled when she started crying. My child was traumatized and I was furious! This happened in the absence of her father. I discovered a week later that trouble was brewing at home.

The following Friday, my ex called to say he wouldn't be picking up the children. His reason seemed a bit odd and I suspected he was covering up something. Saturday evening, he called to tell the children that his phone number had changed. On Sunday, as I was preparing to leave for church, the phone rang again.

"If my wife comes there, please don't let the kids go anywhere near her..." Worried, I warned the children to be on the lookout. In any case, my daughter's story (confirmed by her brother) and my dream were taking on significance. My ex-spouse had remarried shortly after our divorce. The newlyweds, with a new baby, had now separated. Although he was still blaming me for everything that had gone wrong in our marriage, I said a prayer for him. The next time he came to get the children was to take them to his new apartment.

One day he called to tell me not to cash the child support check; he had emergencies. Deciding that I would not help him shoulder the consequences of his foolish choices, I had his wages garnished. It was already on the books from the time of our settlement. I had anticipated such a day as this. Outraged at his audacity and no longer willing to be a doormat or "pin cushion" (his words), I erected new boundaries. By June, I was receiving the check from his employer without being subject to his every whim. He had lost the privilege of considering child support a charitable handout to be reduced or withheld at will.

The children were the only people still under his control. When they were unwilling to go with him, he argued that it was his right to see them (agreed) and that, as the parent, I should "force" them out the door (disagreed). One day I was begging them to "just go" so he would quit leaning on the doorbell. My frayed nerves needed some peace and quiet. Avizi had curled himself around the base of the recliner in protest. Forcing them out the door would have been emotional abandonment. I wouldn't do it.

The man angrily threatened to take me to court. To legally protect myself, I felt compelled to report the incident. I was told that the children were old enough to choose not to go. He dragged me to court anyway. The real reason? His "new hardship"—their baby. With the utmost irritation, I again prepared court papers, wondering when the nightmare would end. The rain was pouring down.

Concern over growing legal debt and my precarious financial status was escalating when I received the call regarding Mama's decline. This was just after Clarissa became my helper. With some financial assistance from my church, I purchased three tickets to Boston.

Before leaving, I kept a doctor's appointment for a physical and was diagnosed with high blood pressure. No surprise. It was October 7th, 1996. We arrived in Boston two days later and celebrated Mama's 79th birthday on October 10th. She died on October 31st, the same day I was scheduled to appear in court.

The hearing was postponed in consideration of my loss, and I switched gears from legal concerns to prepare for a funeral. There were duties to perform and I walked through them like a robot. The rain fell heavily on November 9th, as Mama's casket was lowered into her final resting place. The rain continued as we walked away.

## *WHEN MAMA DIED*

When Mama died, the numbness deepened.
While others wept, my eyes were dry.
It wasn't that I wasn't grieving,
The pain just burrowed deep inside,
Sending my emotions into lockdown.

You'll recall my visit to the doctor in early October. She had made the cursory remark, "Your breasts seem kind of lumpy." I had murmured that they usually felt like that just before my period. The doctor had also reminded me that it was time for my biannual mammogram. Between the trips to Boston, I was placed on a blood pressure medication. So much was happening and the world would not stop spinning to let me off. I mechanically trudged through my daily duties, needing to rest often.

A few weeks after Mama's burial, while showering, I discovered a lump in my right breast. Hoping I was dreaming, I kept checking. "It's a lump all right," I thought. "Wasn't I supposed to be getting a mammogram? Did I ever get the authorization?" My mind was in a fog. I couldn't remember so I called the doctor, then made an appointment for December 5th. All week long I checked and rechecked, hoping the lump wouldn't be there. When I suddenly realized I had missed my period, a friend suggested it was from all the stress.

On December 4th, the children, their father and I met with a mediator in Conciliation Court. I was almost flooded out of my chair by the downpour of acid rain, another toxic shock to my already overburdened spirit. By the end of the session, my head was throbbing. The mediator was not deceived. I felt some relief when she pointed out that if each parent built and maintained a strong relationship with the children, the other would not be able to undermine it. Best of all, the children were heard, and an agreement was reached regarding visitation with which they were comfortable. We were to revisit Conciliation Court in three months to see if the arrangement had been amenable to all.

My mammogram was sandwiched between two days in court. The technician marked the lump, placed my breast on a glass plate, lowered another plate, and kept lowering until the breast core was completely flattened. I winced. She apologized. My first mammogram had been in 1994 and it had been clear. This was my second. Some friends had suggested that the lump was probably benign. One said she had two such lumps removed and they had been benign.

While I waited in the dressing room, the doctor examined the pictures. I was brought back for more X-rays and then ushered into another room for an ultrasound.

"There is definitely something suspicious here," the radiologist muttered, staring at the computer screen. As the technician moved her instrument around my breast. "I will order a biopsy. Call your PCP for the details."

My ex-husband, his mother, and his *new* girlfriend met me in court the following day. How I wished I still had a mother to call for support. For a few fleeting minutes, I chuckled at the case being heard before mine. His tart sense of humor suggested that the judge was burned out on human depravity and folly. Admonishing the plaintiff, the judge suggested that, rather than fight his wife over $10,000 (which he thought was community property but might not be), he would do better to work hard and make himself some money. He listed all the fees the man would have to pay if he pursued the matter, in which case he would probably end up with two bucks. The admonition seemed to fall on deaf ears.

Attempting to minimize my disability, my ex and his lawyer tried to convince the judge that I could get a job anytime. After all, I had homeschooled my children. The adversary even complimented my "very good organizational skills," though it wasn't done for my benefit. Unfortunately, I could not compliment their math skills. By their calculations, $900 a month became $20,000 a year, the alleged income from the job I held 15 years earlier. Perhaps they were adding inflation, you think? Anyway, when the judge questioned me, I set the record straight.

When asked if I had any other physical problems, unwilling to discuss the possibility of cancer, I said "no." After the proceedings, I informed my lawyer about the pending biopsy.

"Why did you say 'no' when the judge asked you about other problems?"

"Because I don't know the result yet. It could be positive or negative. Besides, I don't want to discuss it here."

The judge recognized that we were only in court so child support could be transferred from the older children to the new baby. He was "tired of the primary children being lost in the shuffle." In my favor, he recognized that, as a recipient of disability aid, I would have to declare spousal support as income and therefore lose it. The child support was adjusted accordingly, and my ex was ordered to pay legal fees to my attorney.

There was a lull in the storm that morning. The sun was beginning to break out from behind the dark clouds that had hovered over me for so long. Would I have time to dry out before the next deluge?

## *NARCISSUS*

He majored in self-centeredness
And minored in commitment.
Displaying his charm for others,
He put his best foot forward,
And with the other, kicked his family to the curb.
He fled responsibility to another woman's arms.
She scratched his itch, believing it was love,
But soon discovered he was enamored only with himself.
Now those same arms that caught him as he ran from them,
With one last scratch have thrown him back
Into the pool of his self-absorption.

## YOUR DAUGHTER'S NEED

Can you just take a minute
To step outside your brain?
Can you forget self long enough
To see another's pain?
Then look inside your daughter,
She's just eleven years old,
Yet there's, already in her heart
A void that's deep and cold.

It's a hole shaped like Daddy
That Mama cannot fill,
But your coldness and unkindness
On her love have put a chill.
Can you see the angry turmoil
Your departure has incurred?
Can you feel the deep rejection
From your actions she's inferred?

Don't you think she's deserving
Of some tender, loving words?
Can you forgive her failures,
Especially when you think of yours?
Selfishly you've told her
How much she owes to you,
But how much her Daddy owes her
You just haven't got a clue.

She needs love unconditional,
This darling little girl.
She needs to know she's special,
That she's Daddy's little pearl.
Do not blame your defects
On this precious child,
For if you were more loving,
To see you she'd be wild.

153

But if she shrinks from seeing you,
Then you need to look again
At the things that you've been doing
To cause her heart such pain.
If you live to be an old man,
You may need her love and care;
That's why she thinks about you
And keeps you in her prayers.

# FORGIVENESS IS A CHOICE

As a young girl, I learned that my significance would come from serving and pleasing men, but felt uneasy with the idea. The Bible does command a woman to submit to her husband, but God's commands are for our betterment, never for our detriment. Submission does not diminish her value in any way. She should never be forced to submit through emotional, verbal or physical abuse.

Scripture exhorts all of us to submit to one another out of reverence for Christ (Ephesians 5:21). A husband is commanded to love his wife sacrificially, and as he loves his own body (Ephesians 5:25). This was casually mentioned during wedding ceremonies, while the command for women to submit was constantly reiterated. Despite my disquiet, I internalized the message that, to be a good Christian girl or woman, I must unequivocally submit to men. "Don't rock the boat" and all would be well.

Growing up under authoritarian rule, I was denied freedom of expression. Repressed and frustrated, I was unable to vent my emotions in a healthy way and developed the bad habit of blaming myself when there was interpersonal conflict. If the conflict was with an adult, as the child, I couldn't win. In my marriage, I negated personal needs and desires in order to please. Any assertiveness was met with resentment and subtle reminders that I wouldn't win. Frequent head-trips and putdowns left me feeling diminished and unloved. My spouse wasn't always unkind, but that was the problem; the striking inconsistencies kept me baffled and unsure.

I don't know if he was always conscious of the impact of his actions, but he once advised me, "Protect yourself." When I began to protect myself, when my "no" became stronger, my spouse ramped up the control. I loved him but learned that love has limits; tough love sets limits, the only possible way to save the relationship. Erecting boundaries was new for me; if I tried to present them in a congenial manner, I was not taken seriously. I had to literally and figuratively scream my protest. When my spouse understood the boundaries were here to stay, he defected.

Though we met often to discuss reconciliation, even with counselors, he remained unwilling to acknowledge my pain. According to him, "The relationship is important but your emotions are not." I was tired of trying to legitimize my existence. He said he was searching for truth. I think, in fact, he was running from it.

Thank God for friends, pastors and counselors who kept me centered during this challenging season. There were enough of them to shield me from the criticism of ignorant meddlers. When the need for relief from pain drew me toward denial, friends brought me back to reality, reminding me that I was not accountable for my spouse or his choices. My responsibility was to protect myself and my children.

I confess my contribution to the marital conflict via my own dysfunctions and sinful responses. One thing was certain: I loved the man and was faithful to him. I wanted to save our marriage, but couldn't do it alone. Sadly, the marriage crashed and burned, failing to reflect God's enduring love to those who were watching. None of us escaped unscathed and my distress was intensified by the children's pain.

Jesus said we should forgive those who mistreat us, but this does not preclude erecting boundaries against another's sin. Some say "forgive and forget," but I need not forget in order to forgive. The danger in forgetting is that I may allow an abusive act to be repeated. I understand that to be completely healed, I must completely forgive. Recovery takes time, but eventually, the pain of remembering will diminish.

Anger is a signal that all is not well, and there are actions for which righteous anger is justified. The Bible, however, exhorts, "In your anger do not sin..." (Ephesians 4:26). Pretending I have no anger will only drive it underground, not remove it. Recognizing that bitterness will only imprison me in the pain of the past, I choose to rid myself of anger.

I learned that forgiveness is a process. The deeper the wound, the harder the process. It is like peeling an onion, layer by layer, each layer revealing deeper hurt and evoking more tears. To truly forgive, I must understand the cost of the wrong perpetrated against me. I cannot thoroughly forgive until I have accurately assessed the extent of the injury. Then, in light of the mercy granted me by God for my greater offenses against Him, I choose to extend mercy to my offender (Ephesians 4:32). An unforgiving spirit can never be a free spirit. I want to be free from bitterness, so I must depend on God's strength to complete the process.

It is my sole responsibility to offer forgiveness whether or not the offender seeks it. God commands it. Reconciliation, however, can only happen if there is a change of heart and both parties pursue it. Forgiving someone does not mean allowing him to continue harming me.

Joseph was sold into slavery by his Hebrew brothers. After much suffering, he became Prince of Egypt. During a famine, his brothers went to Egypt for food. Joseph knew them, but they did not recognize him. He had already forgiven them, yet had not forgotten their betrayal. Hiding his identity, Joseph evaluated his brothers' dispositions through a series of tests. When their remorse was evident, Joseph revealed himself, embracing his brothers in reconciliation (Genesis 37:11-36; 42:8; 45:15).

Unfortunately, my story did not end in reconciliation. When the changing seasons of life thrust the realities of my divorce to the forefront, I choose to forgive. When I recall the betrayal, I choose to forgive. When the hurt and pain resurface, I choose to forgive. It is in the process of forgiving that I am freed to pursue and find joy.

"See to it that no one misses the grace of God and that no bitter root grows up to cause trouble and defile many." Hebrews 12:15

## HELP ME FORGIVE

Lord, drain the pain out of my heart,
Let not bitterness be rooted there.
Pour down Your love on smoldering grudge
And still the breeze that fans the flames of hate.
Help me forgive as I have been forgiven,
Bringing to Earth a little taste of Heaven.

"Forgive us our debts as we also have forgiven our debtors." Matthew 6:12

## FORGIVING GOD

Me forgiving God?
What a preposterous thought!
What wrong has He done?
Requests not granted
Lead me to believe He failed.
My misconception!
He always answers:
"Yes, no, wait," or, "I will give
Better than you ask.
Forgive and be free
From internal corrosion
That blocks joy's entrance."
Forgiveness is me,
Releasing all bitterness,
Receiving God's grace.

*Joy Walker*

## CLEANSE ME

Cleanse my feeble mind, dear Lord,
From every thought of sin;
Fill it with Your Holy Word,
Enthrone Yourself within.
Help me set my thoughts on
Things just and pure and true,
Things lovely and of good report,
The virtues found in You.
May I in thinking, Lord, of You,
So learn Your perfect will,
That men may in my actions see
The God who in me dwells.

# PART 9. UNWELCOME INTRUDER

## THE DIAGNOSIS

On December 11<sup>th</sup>, 1996, I was sipping hot tea in a room at the Diagnostic Imaging Center. The technician, having just done my ultrasound, had asked me to wait for the doctor's feedback.

"Hi, I'm Dr. Brown!" Shaking my hand, he explained, "It seems you have a cluster of cysts in the right breast. There are also cysts in the left breast." He was scanning the films. "Since they weren't there when you did your first mammogram in '94, we'll watch them. You don't want a biopsy if you don't have to, do you?"

"No," I muttered, unsure.

"Then come back in six months and we'll see if there are any changes." I felt no relief and was very depressed all weekend. Maybe I knew in my spirit that it wasn't really over, or maybe it was the letdown from the other emotional storms. My Sunday school classmates expressed their relief when I shared the news.

The following Monday afternoon, December 16<sup>th</sup>, the phone rang. "This is Dr. Gooden from the lab where you came for a biopsy last Wednesday. A team of radiologists looked at your ultrasound, and all agree that you should return for a biopsy. There is a form of micro-invasive cancer that starts in the ducts. Looks like it's just starting to leave the ducts, so with luck we'll catch it early. Someone will call you to make an appointment."

There was a slight disturbance in my spirit, then numbness settled in. Preparing to leave home for the lab on December 18<sup>th</sup>, I felt a swell behind my eyes. Tears were gathering reinforcement. Unable to weather a deluge right then, I kept them at bay. My spirit somehow knew there would be pouring down of heavy rain again.

As I exchanged information with the receptionist, the technician approached the counter. She was a soft-spoken woman who had done my ultrasound the previous week.

"You are back?"

"They told me to come back for the biopsy."

"Bummer!"

Local anesthesia was applied to my right breast as it dangled through a hole in the table. The only discomfort came from having to lie perfectly still for about two hours. I could hear what sounded like a staple gun, and could feel a dull sensation as if the doctor was shooting my breast full of staples. He was doing a needle core biopsy. What sounded like a gun was the instrument used to close the needle over the tissue being removed for testing. I learned later that they had inserted five needles, to which even the surgeon said, "Ouch," on reading the report.

As I walked out of the lab numb and dazed, someone said, "Merry Christmas!" I thought, "That's right, it's almost Christmas." I felt like answering, "Bah, humbug!"

Working obsessively all next day, I finished the last six lessons of a Braille reading correspondence course I had been working on. Then the ominous phone call came.

"...I'm afraid we found some malignancy. I think we are catching it early. Dr. Mahoney will be contacting you about the next step. I'd say you could safely wait 'til the first of the year, but I wouldn't wait much longer. I'm sorry to deliver this kind of news just before Christmas."

Incredulous, I called friends and family, repeating the news in monotone as if sharing information about someone else. It was December 19th. "I knew I'd been falling apart," I said to my sister, "but I didn't expect cancer."

I don't know what prompted me to ask the question, but when I last saw Mama, I asked the doctor if he had checked her for cancer. Unsure of the cause of her pain, he had suggested exploratory surgery, but Daddy had declined. At Mama's funeral, I discovered that one of my cousins had died from cancer. I didn't know then that the disease had already taken root in me.

Doug, the Sunday school teacher, read a note from me to the class:

"...It seems that I'm being launched into yet another period of testing. I would like to bow out or pass the honor on to someone else, but I do not have a choice (chuckles). I was just diagnosed with breast cancer (gasps). I am very scared about the unknown, but must still believe Romans 8:28 and Jeremiah 29:11. I need your prayers and support more than ever."

The silence was broken by Doug's voice. "But you told us last week…" After I explained the recent events, he led the class in prayer. Several people hugged me, expressing their sympathy. Some were crying. I still had not cried.

The Monday before Christmas, accompanied by my friend Judy, I had my first consultation with the surgeon.

Dr. Carlson remarked as he entered the room, "You are so young!"

"I'm 48," I replied, not thinking it that young.

"Even so, I'm used to seeing women in their 50's and 60's." He gave me two weeks to decide between a lumpectomy with radiation and a mastectomy with chemotherapy. I cringed at the thought of either scenario. My friend, Roslyn, had done some research on my behalf and had copied excerpts from *Reclaiming Your Health* by John Robbins. He discussed the negative long-term effects of chemo and radiation; i.e., damage to tissue causing growth of secondary cancers in other parts of the body. I was against radiation immediately. Glancing at the information I handed him, the surgeon tried to assure me.

"The radiation beam would only be aimed at your breast and would not affect any major organs except those in the chest."

"But my lungs and heart are in my chest!"

"I know, but the amount of radiation is minimal. You may get a sunburn, or at worst develop a cough that will eventually go away."

"Would you consider a lumpectomy without radiation?"

"If that is what you want, you will have to go somewhere else. It is too risky. I won't do it!"

The shock was intensifying. After collecting some informational brochures, I left the office carrying a mountain on my back. It was true. I had cancer, and it wasn't going away.

# CHRISTMAS BLESSINGS

"Friends are there when you need them."

In our house, the Christmas tree was decorated right after Thanksgiving. My son's birthday is in December, so he got to enjoy the decorations for an entire month. The tradition continued for Christmas '96, though I was not in a celebratory mood. The recent traumas had left me in a stupor. I didn't have a spouse at home to pick up the slack, but I kept functioning somehow.

After Mama's death and the legal proceedings, I had dared to think, "Surely there'll be a respite from grief now. Maybe I'll start fresh after Christmas." I had hoped that the New Year would be the one in which I could focus on Joy. Now I would indeed be focusing on me, but not in the manner I had anticipated. Physically and emotionally drained, I couldn't cope with all the demands.

Gradually I absorbed the fact that my life would never be the same. The "D" word loomed large on the horizon. No one knows how long they have to live, but a cancer diagnosis surely brings the issue to the forefront, and every time I watched television there was some new story about cancer.

Although I was mostly in shock during the Christmas season, there were moments when humor brought needed relief. With my daughter's help, I composed "Zap the Boobs" and "Mastectomy Song." In the process, I had subconsciously made my decision to have a mastectomy. This decision was later confirmed by second and third opinions.

On Christmas morning, our pastor surprised us with a gift from the church. It was heartwarming to know that people cared. The children had a brief visit from their father, after which we left for a friend's house.

A couple from church invited us to spend Christmas Day with their family. The day was pleasant, though I remember being very weary. I chatted with everyone from Karla's rocking chair, dozing off occasionally. The children were in a constant uproar, chasing each other with water guns, dashing in and out of the house until

Randy, who had three boys, put a stop to it. We felt like part of the family. Karla even had a gift for each of us. I was particularly pleased that the children were enjoying themselves. I couldn't have kept them entertained had we remained at home, and they did not need to be burdened with my preoccupations.

That evening, I received a call from Hyacinth, who had planned to spend the next day with us. She asked me what I needed. I suggested things the children would enjoy. Hyacinth arrived carrying a huge basket of fruit, a freshly-baked chocolate cake, and leftovers from her Christmas dinner. After we visited for a while, she asked the kids, "Where would you like to go for lunch?" They chorused almost in unison, "Jack in the Box!" There was one within walking distance.

After the children left with their dad, Hyacinth and I went shopping. I was moved by her kindness, but a little uncomfortable. Shopping without weighing the cost of each item was foreign to me. She even took me to the local health food store to purchase vitamins. As she prepared to leave, I thanked her profusely.

"This is such a blessing! I really do appreciate it. We will enjoy everything. This is so much more than I expected."

"Well, it was my pleasure, and thank you for allowing me to bless you!"

Hyacinth has continued to be supportive on many levels, and I consider her a friend indeed. The road ahead would be bumpy, but I was not alone.

## MASTECTOMY SONG
(Tune: "Oh Hanukkah Oh Hanukkah")

Lumpectomy, mastectomy, which one will it be?
See how the surgeons are dancing with glee,
Gathered 'round the table at sight of this treat,
Waving their scalpels as if I am fresh meat;
And while they are dancing, one surgeon is bending low,
Brandishing a knife he is standing on my right
And my poor boob it will have to go!

## ZAP THE BOOBS
(Tune: "Deck the Halls")

Zap the boobs with radiation.
Refrain: Fa la la la la la la la la ouch!
Or slice them off with great precision. (Refrain)
Where'll the surgeon place the incision? (Refrain)
I must make this grave decision. (Refrain)


## CANCER PRAYER

The diagnostic shock had come,
Fear had left my heart quite numb,
I'm thawing now and pain runs deep,
Terror too invades my sleep.

Jesus, I put my trust in Thee,
There's so much I cannot see,
Yet I know I must believe
If of these fears I'd be relieved.

This new and dread reality
Makes me face my mortality;
Makes me wonder what's ahead
And how soon I may be dead.

The fog is heavy on my brain,
My stomach tightens in its pain.
I need Your strength to see me through,
Oh Lord God, do I need You!

# OPINIONS AND DECISIONS

"Breast cancer never kills anyone; it's the complications that do. Removing your breast would reduce the chance of recurrence."

The radiation oncologist was attempting to allay my fears, but I was not convinced. If breast cancer kills no one, why do I keep hearing about the thousands of women who die each year? Tell me there are survivors, but don't tell me breast cancer kills no one. I have a friend whose sister, only 29 years old, died a year after her mastectomy. The point was, nobody knew how much cancer was in my body or if it had already spread; nobody knew if I would be a survivor. My fears were real! Having a body part removed was a traumatic consideration. Would I die? What about my children? I begged God for at least seven years so both children would have graduated high school.

A few days later, I was in another doctor's office seeking a third opinion.

"I would recommend a mastectomy followed by chemotherapy. If the cancer is hormone-positive, I could put you on the oral medication Tamoxifen for five years. When do you want to do it?"

His abrupt approach shocked me! I could scarcely take in the reality that my breast would have to be cut off, and he wanted me to set an appointment then and there. His insensitivity appalled me. It was all in a day's work for him. For me, it was a harrowing, life-changing decision. I returned to the first surgeon.

Roslyn introduced me to The Wellness Community. It is a non-profit organization providing (free of charge) support groups, medical resources and psycho-social supportive services for cancer patients. I attended my first breast cancer networking group the first weekend in January 1997.

Intrigued and terrified, I listened to women tell their stories of diagnosis and treatment. It was reassuring to share my fears with people who understood and validated all my emotions. On the other hand, I was alarmed to hear that some women had received chemotherapy, radiation and Tamoxifen—all three. I had believed that these were either/or choices. One woman had written her will before her surgery. I needed to do that, but was already too traumatized for such an undertaking.

The following week, I attended an orientation meeting, met other cancer survivors, and made plans to join a weekly support group. Fern, also a cancer patient, agreed to pick me up on her way from work if I joined a Wednesday group. I offered to have dinner ready as a trade-off for transportation.

A young woman from the networking group called me a few days later with information about a naturopathic doctor. Roslyn had also been researching alternative treatments on my behalf. Both had my best interest in mind, but alternative medicine was a costly venture, not at all compatible with my meager budget. I had been reading too. It seemed that, despite the stories and claims of miracle cures, there were survivors as well as casualties on both sides. Whatever the treatment of choice, God is the one who ultimately decides who lives or dies.

I had to be sensible. With two children who needed me, I was not free to focus only on my needs. There was no point in starting something I couldn't finish. My HMO would cover conventional treatment. I could add vitamin and herbal supplementation along with basic changes to my diet. Although the naturopath offered some good dietary advice, he disapproved of letting them cut off my breast. I felt pressured. I didn't think that my life situation afforded me any other options.

Reconstructive surgery was my next consideration, whether or not to have it, when to do it, and what kind. Beverley, a support group member, chose a procedure called the Tran flap. Her own abdominal tissue was used to reconstruct the breast during her mastectomy. She made this choice to avoid the jolt of waking up without a body part. It was major surgery, and she spent several days in intensive care.

Beverley advised me to seriously consider my options. I could choose to have an implant done at the time of the mastectomy, or forego reconstruction altogether and wear a prosthesis. I considered the mastectomy sufficient invasion and settled on wearing a prosthesis. I could change my mind later. There was a law that prohibited medical providers from denying a woman that choice.

Wanting to make informed decisions, I obtained several talking books from the Braille Institute library. What I heard so unnerved me, I could hardly summon the strength to turn the tape over. I just lay there dazed. The reality was that nobody really knew how this saga would end. The unknown was so frightening! I was not in control. Apart from moments of angry outbursts, I was mostly numb. I read a book by Betty Roland, *First You Cry*, but I couldn't cry for a long time.

Of all the breast cancer survivors I had met, no two people had the same response or treatment profile. There were so many variables: the stage of cancer ranging from one to four (four being the most dangerous), the size of the tumor, and the type of cancer. It could be invasive or non-invasive, ER-positive or HER2-negative. The outcome differed if the woman was post or pre-menopausal, if the cancer had already metastasized to the lymph nodes, and according to the number of lymph nodes involved. Trying to decide what to do based on what someone else had done was mind-boggling.

On January 20th, I returned to the first surgeon. Having read somewhere that the best time for surgery was 12 to 16 days after my last menstrual cycle, I planned accordingly. The date was set for January 28th.

I had a page of questions for Dr. Carlson. He was impressed that I had done my research, and said I probably knew more than he did. That was not at all comforting. It seemed surgeons just concern themselves with cutting things out or off. He couldn't answer very many questions about what would come next. I commented that the surgeon working on my hand may not have a clue about what's wrong with my toe. He added (half in jest) that modern medicine is so specialized that, for my toe, I might need three specialists: a neurologist, a podiatrist and an orthopedist. Whatever happened to the family doctor who understood all the dynamics that affect a person's health?

I remember asking a doctor at a seminar if cancer and stress were related. He answered "no" without hesitation. I was taken aback. Much of my reading had pointed out a strong correlation. I learned that everyone has some cancer cells in their body, but a healthy immune system is usually able to destroy them. Excess stress compromises the immune system, rendering it ineffective against the rapidly reproducing cancer cells. It was noteworthy that many cancer survivors had been experiencing one or more major traumatic life events just before their diagnosis. While I understand that genetic and other environmental factors contribute to cancer, I still do not comprehend a doctor's refusal to admit that stress plays a major role.

Once the date for surgery was set, I made arrangements for the children. Eleanor, a school mom, agreed to keep them for the days I would be hospitalized. She would take care of getting them to school. Next, I had to decide who would help me after surgery. A friend, whose daughter was about the same age as mine, would stay with me the first weekend after surgery. The church offered to pay a live-in caregiver for the following week. My Sunday school class would be providing meals. Now, I just needed to get my house in order.

The phone kept ringing. So many people cared and wanted me to know I was in their thoughts and prayers. With a great support team in place and major decisions settled, I was as ready as I'd ever be for January 28th, 1997.

## DOES MAMA SEE?

A few days before my mastectomy, I dreamed of Mama for the first time since her death. There were a series of shelves attached to the wall opposite my bed. On the very top shelf, Mama laid, face down. Daddy and Faith entered the room, caught sight of her and became greatly concerned that the shelf would give way and Mama would fall.

Mama's body seemed as thin and feeble as it was during her illness, but to our surprise, she began to raise her upper torso. As she did, blood flowed from her chest. The dream ended.

## BREAST PAIN

One struggle after another came:
Rejection, divorce, the legal game,
The funeral that laid hope to rest,
The heightened grief within my breast,
The pain of children's thwarted dreams,
The prayers ignored by God, it seems,
My mother's suffering, hard and long,
Her body weak reduced to bones.

The doubts, the questioning of God,
Life's riddles still not understood,
The feeling that I cannot cope,
The sliding down the slippery slope
Unable to turn back the clock
Wishing my spinning world would stop
Let me off to catch my breath
Heal hurts solidifying in my breast.

I would let go of all this pain,
This pouring down of heavy rain,
This fierce erosion of my heart,
This lewd attack on body part,
This fear that fires up my brain
Then leaves me numb like Novocain.
My mother's gone, her suffering done,
While I with cancer must fight on.

My bosom heaves again today:
"Thy will be done, Dear Lord," I say.
"Though breast may fall from surgeon's knife,
It's You, O God, who guards my life;
And if You will for me to live,
Then strength enough I know You'll give
Through struggles that may still remain,
For in them all, You'll be the same." (Day of mastectomy)

## *VISION*

I don't need 20/20 vision
To see my body's mutilation,
To understand a part of me is gone.
Each time I wash or dress or move,
The pain, the wound is there to prove
The permanent absence of my breast
And to raise questions about the rest.
Then there are the unpleasant rumors
About the presence of more tumors.
Perhaps they'll go on cutting
Until there is nothing.

I do need spiritual vision
To get past my mutilation,
To see that who I am is still intact.
The tears will wash my spirit clean.
On God I'll simply have to lean.
His plan is best, though still unknown.
I will submit until it's shown.
And even if they go on cutting,
Of me there never will be nothing,
For when they lay my body down
Somewhere six feet beneath the ground,
My spirit will have gone up higher,
Released at last from suffering's fire.

"So we do not lose heart. Though our outer self is wasting away, our inner self is being renewed day by day." 2 Corinthians 4:16

# CANCER NEWS

March 15, 1997

Dear Friends and Well-wishers,

"...Have you not heard? The Lord is the everlasting God, the Creator of the ends of the earth. He will not grow tired or weary, and his understanding no one can fathom. He gives strength to the weary and increases the power of the weak." Isaiah 40:28, 29

Praise be to God for His immeasurable grace, and thanks to you who have allowed yourselves to be used for the outpouring of His love and mercy on my children and me.

I recently had a modified radical mastectomy. The diagnosis of breast cancer came as a shock just before Christmas and shortly after my mother's death. She died on October 31st, after a prolonged illness. During that time, I was also embroiled in a legal battle with my ex-spouse. From my perspective, the timing could not have been worse. I was already in so much pain. As I struggled through a wide range of emotions, and, in an attempt to understand the "why" of it all, I read two particularly relevant books: *Where Is God When It Hurts* by Philip Yancey, and *When God Makes No Sense* by Dr. James Dobson. Here is what I either learned or was reminded of.

God cared enough about me to send His Son Jesus to die for my sins so that I can have a right relationship with Him. He has proven that His love for me is everlasting, and His plan for me is good (Jeremiah 31:3; 29:11). While He is a tender, compassionate God, His plan for us involves more than just our present comfort. As we become more aware that our sojourn here is temporary, we will understand and accept that the larger scope of His concern is in the refinement of our souls.

He is equipping me for eternity in His presence and will use all of life's circumstances to make me a better person on the inside where it counts most. If my finite mind could grasp all of who God is, or understand all that He does, He would no longer be God. I must therefore trust Him to work all things together for my good (Romans 8:28). I was also reminded that, without trials, we would never know the triumph of joy, and, without affliction, we would never cultivate perseverance. It is my response to suffering that determines whether I become bitter or better.

Your generosity (prayers, phone calls, cards, letters, gifts, meals, visits...) has been a beautiful reflection of God's love and care for me. I still need your prayers. The cancer has spread to the lymph nodes, making further treatment necessary. The surgeon removed 15 lymph nodes and eight had cancer. Yes, chemotherapy and radiation sound scary, but I am sure that nothing (not even cancer) can separate me from the love of God which is in Christ Jesus (Romans 8:38, 39). I am confident that He will bring me through this too.

Shortly after surgery, I received a Communications Award for my poetry from the Braille Institute. As a part-time student, I have been learning to use a talking computer, hoping to acquire one soon with a view toward publishing another book of poems.

The children are doing well. Both have been little troopers. We are no longer homeschooling. Avizi will graduate eighth grade from our church school in June. Agalia is presently in fifth grade at the local elementary school. My son was bragging this morning that he is already taller than me; his sister is not far behind. Single-parenting is tough, but my children are precious and worth the effort.

Again, my deepest thanks to all of you for your support.

Sincerely,

Joy


## *LET GOD BE GOD*

If God were foolish and fickle enough
To be easily manipulated,
Any attempt to depend on Him
Would be utterly frustrated.

If He were wishy-washy enough
To give us whatever we requested,
How could His promise to keep us from harm
Or His wisdom and guidance be trusted?

Were He to hold grudges as some of us do,
Unwilling to pardon offenders,
Not one of us ever would taste of His love,
For we all fall short of His standards.
If God did not have our best interest in mind,
He wouldn't send trials to improve us.
He'd let us escape all the tests of life,
Then on a shelf, useless, would leave us.

The Potter knows best how to handle the clay,
How to break it and bend it and knead it,
How best to remove imperfections He sees
Before sculpting a vessel of beauty.
So let God be God—the Creator All-Wise,
Omnipotent, Trustworthy, Loving!
Let us kneel before Him to worship in awe
And reverence the One who is Sovereign!


## WHICH ONE ARE YOU?

Some people hide to nurse their wounds,
Some want to talk to ease the pain,
Some glibly ask, "How do you do?"
Then quickly leave without a clue.
Some shun the ones who're hurting now
To wait till they have better days,
Some act with genuine concern,
Aware tomorrow may be their turn.
Which one are you?

Some say, "Call when you need to talk,
But please don't call me if I'm tired,
Or, if my favorite soap is on,
You'll have to wait until I'm done."
Some say, "I'm glad to be of help,
Do call again if you need more!"
Some say, "You've had sufficient grace,
So why are you back in my face?"
Which one are you?

Some people don't reach out for fear
They'll be rebuffed, looked down upon,
Some have been wounded when they've asked,
Been made to feel like second class.
Some folk are too proud to receive
From others when they have a need,
Some are aware that gifts of love
Are truly sent from God above.
Which one are you?

Some help but not with motive pure,
Some turn their heads and walk on by,
Some jump right in where there's a need,
Good Samaritans who roll up their sleeves
To give the help that's relevant,
Ready to serve at every chance,
Knowing that giving to the poor
Is simply honoring the Lord.
Which one are you?

## *WHY BOTHER?*

Yesterday you asked as you passed
(As if you cared) how I was,
Without stopping to hear me say
"I'm feeling down."
You never even turned around
As you quickly walked away.
Today you stop to ask how I am.
My answer is quite real:
"I'm feeling blue…"
You retort before I'm through:
"Don't feel that way,
Everything will be okay!"
These words I ponder,
At your insensitivity wonder.
You keep right on talking
While I go on hurting.
"Have a good day!" you say
As again you walk away.

## LOOK GOOD, FEEL BETTER

Two months after the mastectomy, I attended a workshop
sponsored by The American Cancer Society and held at The
Wellness Community. Created to help women minimize the effects
of cancer treatment on their physical appearance, "Look Good, Feel
Better" started with a video. Women of varying ages shared how the
workshop had given them options. They didn't have to look bad on
the outside even when feeling lousy on the inside.

Makeup tips were demonstrated for replacing missing eyebrows
and eyelashes, and for covering up skin blemishes caused by the
ravages of chemotherapy. Each woman received a bag of makeup,
generously donated by several cosmetic companies and worth around
$200. I was timid about exposing my ignorance, but my friend,

Pamela, quickly told me what everything was. There were also wigs, hats, turbans and scarves that could be used to disguise hair loss and maintain a look of femininity.

A licensed cosmetologist volunteered her time to run the workshop. Remarking on how blemish-free my skin was, she requested the use of my face for the demonstration. With her coaching, I actually put mascara on for the first time. Would I ever be able to do it on my own? Making myself look like a clown was not very appealing, so I thought it best not to try. I might poke my eyes out and blind myself further. For the moment, I giggled at the other women's "oohs" and "aahs." This was fun for a while and did take our minds off of cancer temporarily.

Trying on the wigs was even more entertaining. I told my kids I would get a long, blond wig. Avizi said that if I did, I would have to let him pierce his ears. I selected three wigs: a shoulder-length dirty blond with pageboy cut and bangs; a crew cut dark auburn; and a short, curly light auburn. I also selected various hats and colorful scarves. Since I was all made up, I decided to wear the dark auburn wig home.

A few hours after returning home, I lost my joy. The reason for the workshop suddenly hit me. I knew it would take great effort to bother with any of this on the days when chemo would be taking its toll. Crying for a while, I wiped mascara along with the tears. One thing I knew, makeup was not going to inhibit my crying. I put Braille labels on the cosmetics for easy identification. This way, I could play with them when no one was looking.

Agalia, now 11 years old, became my beautician and had fun making her Mama look pretty. Next morning, with her help, I donned the curly wig, applied some makeup and went to church. A friend approached me smiling.

"Hi, my name is Kelly!" She pretended to be meeting me for the first time.

"Nice to meet you! I'm the new kid on the block!" I giggled. "I'm trying out my new look in preparation for chemotherapy."

Avizi had spent Saturday night with a friend and saw me for the first time at church. He did not look happy.

"Mom! What did you do to your hair?" He was so serious, I couldn't help chuckling. "Come on, Mom! What did you do?" He felt the color made me look old and did not like his mother looking old. I think he wanted to put me in "time-out." That night, both kids giggled as they tried on the wigs, arguing about who would wear which one come next Halloween. I supposed I was as ready as I would ever be to face chemo.

## BIRTHDAY JOY

On April 7th, I visited my surgeon to arrange the surgical placement of a Groshong catheter in my chest. My "roll-away veins" presented a challenge to technicians who wanted my blood. The implantation of this subcutaneous catheter would facilitate delivery of the chemo drugs. Surgery was scheduled for the following Wednesday. Thanks to my friend, Fanny, I was able to go directly from the surgeon's office to the lab for my preoperative blood work.

When we arrived at the hospital two days later, I was in good spirits, knowing God would take care of me as always. Since my reaction to general anesthesia at the time of the mastectomy was severe, I opted for local sedation.

"I already did it at the lab on Monday," I protested as a nurse's aide approached me for another blood draw. She checked, then returned, insisting it had to be done; she couldn't find the lab results. I sustained my protest. Shortly thereafter, another nurse apologized. She had found the report. It sure pays to be assertive.

In the recovery room, the nurse explained that the pain in my left shoulder, neck and arm was probably due to my position during surgery. She suggested I try Tylenol for relief. I spent the next few days mostly in bed, in considerable pain. A nurse suggested stronger medication. Hesitant to have more drugs pumped into my body, I settled on Tylenol.

My Mexican twin, Casandra, paid me a visit. We share a birthday, but are as unalike as spinach and doughnuts.

"Joy, I really want to do something for you, so I was thinking…"

"You thinking? A dangerous thing!"

"Oh, stop it! How about we have a birthday party together? We'll have it at my place. I'll do the cooking and you just invite some friends. All you have to do is eat, have fun, and go home when you're done. I will do the cleaning up."

I chuckled, "So, you're a poet now?" Well, if you put it that way, let me think about it. I'll call a few friends and see what happens."

On my 49th birthday, I awoke with excruciating pain radiating from my chest towards my neck. The pain came with every breath and felt as if someone had a stranglehold on my throat. It was scary, but I intended to enjoy my special day. After a dose of Tylenol, I went about my business. I was enjoying lunch with Ellen when the pain began to bother me again.

Not wanting to leave all the party preparations to Casandra, I picked up a few items from Trader Joe's. Friends had also promised to bring food. There was a special excitement about the spontaneity of this party. I didn't have a chance to get burned out on planning and preparation, wondering if everything would turn out right.

The evening was cool, so I wore my "Tina Turner" wig, dubbed so by my daughter. It was styled in a pageboy, shoulder length with bangs and was dirty blond, if you can imagine. I went all out on makeup with help from my friend, Chris. As I walked downstairs, everybody cheered, "You look great!" All evening long they kept badgering me for a song and dance.

"Look!" I said, giving myself airs. "I do not entertain on my birthday. You should be entertaining me!" I was having a splendid time. Cards with heartfelt wishes and delightful gifts reminded me I was loved.

Throughout the evening, the pain kept rearing its ugly head. I wondered if anyone noticed me clutching at my chest intermittently. Not wanting to be a party pooper, and because I was having such a good time, I managed to hold out until midnight, then retired upstairs. I was awakened by the pain at 4:30AM. Thinking I was having a heart attack, I called for help. The nurse suggested I go to the emergency room immediately.

Hearing the music downstairs, I called Casandra to see if her brother would drive me to the hospital, but he was already gone. Hesitant to bother anyone else at that hour, I took a high dose of Motrin and went back to sleep. A few hours later, the pain jerked me awake again. I located the doctor and called Pamela, who lived close to me. We were on our way to the ER by 8:30AM.

An EKG and chest X-ray were completed before I was wheeled away to another room. I was assured it would be "much quieter." The wait was torturous. Besides the anxiety about my own condition, I had the dubious privilege of listening to the grisly details of the patients on both sides of my bed. Separated only by a curtain, I missed nothing.

An elderly woman had Alzheimer's. Her response, when questioned, confirmed it. On the other side was a man who had been having diarrhea and vomiting for several days. Across the way was a screaming baby who just went on and on. Add the constant bleeping of the monitors to the fact that I hadn't slept much the previous night. In spite of my woes, I couldn't help chuckling when someone asked the baby if he was laughing or crying. He seemed to alternate between the two for variety. The doctor was offering the man with diarrhea some crackers. He wanted to see what would happen to the crackers after they entered his gastrointestinal tract. I hoped it wouldn't happen right there next to me. We already had enough variations on sound effects.

Crackers sounded good to me. I was famished and remembered I was missing the ladies' annual spring luncheon right at that moment. Plucking up some courage, I asked for crackers when the nurse brought some for my neighbor. In the meantime, I speculated that the nurse who had promised me water a few moons before was still digging the well.

Soon someone handed me a paper cup with a nasty tasting liquid which she called a "gastric cocktail." I wondered momentarily if it had come from the man next door. This was supposed to relieve the pain if it had originated from gastric malfunction. It didn't help.

Several hours later, "Doc" still hadn't shown up. They were communicating with him via telephone. He was undoubtedly savoring coffee and doughnuts while I lay starving. A young technician was apologizing profusely as she, like all the others, repeatedly stabbed me in an attempt to draw blood. When would my ordeal end?

Pamela had been gone for a few hours to run errands, so I was all alone in my misery. A doctor I hadn't seen before assured me that my heart and lungs were fine. The pain seemed to be from a musculoskeletal source, probably due to the change in my anatomy and the trauma to which my body had been subjected during my recent surgeries. To add insult to injury, I was then stabbed in my posterior, with an assurance that the medicine thus administered would relieve my pain.

I was still hurting when I returned home. Fortunately, I wasn't at the hospital long enough to hear the gruesome fate of my roommate's crackers. That was a good thing; it was lunch time and I was very hungry. My darling daughter and her friend, Leilani, had cleaned the kitchen and prepared lunch, a pleasant surprise. The next day was April 13th, the six-year anniversary of being dumped by my husband. For once, the memory didn't seem particularly grievous. I was simply happy to be alive.

## BLESSINGS IN BOSTON

I called my father, crying, "Daddy, I can't do this..." Before I could finish the sentence, I was rushing to the bathroom to throw up again. The first dose of Adriamycin, the "red devil," set my throat and esophagus on fire. I hurt with every swallow. I was scared.

Faith had written a play for the annual church banquet and invited me to participate. She offered to purchase my ticket to Boston for the following weekend. Needing to be with family, I accepted.

"Am I really going to lose my hair?" I asked the oncologist. "I need to see the hairdresser."

"You will be wasting your money," he responded. With that confirmation, I headed for the barber and requested a very short haircut. Fanny and I then went to Mervyn's, where she bought me a hat. When I returned home, Avizi again registered his displeasure.

"Mom, what did you do to your hair? You look like Uncle Danny." I thought it really funny and called my brother. "Hey Danny! Your nephew thinks I resemble you in the head."

I arrived at Boston's Logan Airport on May 2nd. A friendly stewardess escorted me to baggage claim to retrieve my luggage. "My ride is waiting *upstays*," she said in her Bostonian drawl, "so I'll leave you here till your party arrives. Is that alright?"

When no one showed, I called home. Daddy had a medical emergency and was at the hospital. Faith and a friend were on their way. After a tedious wait, Faith claimed me, and we headed home.

Little feet pattered toward the front door as I rang the bell to the old homestead.

"It's Auntie Joy! It's Auntie Joy!" they chorused happily. "Where's Avizi and Agalia?"

"I didn't bring them this time." They seemed momentarily deflated, then their vivacity returned as I cried, "Where's my hug?" I threw my cane and purse on the floor, exchanged hugs and kisses with my niece Joanna and nephews Jeremy and Jonathan, lifting them off the floor. Hugging Carol, I headed for the kitchen, our favorite hangout.

Carol and her husband had separated. She and her three children were now living with Daddy. Faith, my youngest sibling, lived with her son Jamal, within walking distance. I was the first one diagnosed with legal blindness, followed by Faith and Carol. Of my three sisters, I was the only one who had regularly endured severe dysmenorrhea. Now I was the first with cancer. Hopefully I would remain the only one.

Daddy returned from the hospital in good spirits. He owned the three-family house we called home, renting out the first and third floors and living on the second. Daddy had gone downstairs to collect rent. While counting the bills, he realized he was "getting foolish." He kept shuffling the money, unable to count. Putting the cash on the table, he attempted to go upstairs, but couldn't open the door. He almost fell. The tenant, realizing something was wrong, led him to her sofa and called 9-1-1.

"Everything looked strange; the paramedics seemed to have round, shiny heads as if they were from outer space."

"Daddy, have you ever seen someone from outer space?" I queried, amused.

On returning home, Daddy stopped downstairs to collect the money. To his dismay, the woman claimed she had given it to him. He was sure he had left it on her table. Her little daughter told Daddy her mother put the money in her purse. The mother, feigning innocence, brought her purse to show Daddy.

"I can't believe she would try to take advantage of you at a time like this," I remarked. "Just pray she'll get a guilty conscience and 'fess up later. Maybe she just couldn't resist the temptation for some easy cash. But Daddy, you should have someone trustworthy help you collect the rent. This could happen again!"

The woman returned, claiming to have found the money under a sofa cushion. Taking Faith by the hand, she led her downstairs and showed her the bills neatly folded under the cushion.

"I would never cheat your father," she protested with a self-righteous air. "It must have fallen out of his pocket when he was sitting there."

"A likely story," I thought. "All those bills just fell out of his pocket, folded themselves and climbed under a cushion in one neat pile. We really gonna believe that one!"

We were chatting and laughing when Daddy announced he had been "a-courting." It seemed a bit outrageous because Mama hadn't even been gone a year.

"So, Daddy," I probed, pretending to be serious, "What's the big rush?"

"I am getting old," he exclaimed good-naturedly.

"Daddy, you been old for some time now. You're 77, remember?" Everyone howled with laughter. We soon grew tired and Daddy drove Faith, Jamal and me to Faith's house.

Faith and I went on a modest shopping spree the following afternoon. I purchased an ensemble for the banquet. It consisted of a black tank top, an ankle-length skirt and long-sleeved jacket in a paisley pattern of black, purple and gold. To top it off, I borrowed Faith's black and gold pillbox hat. I believe I looked rather elegant!

At the banquet, many were surprised and pleased to see me. It was good to be among my people again. After a pleasant meal, we were entertained by a women's trio from New York, followed by Faith's play, in the form of a talk show. The topic was "In whom or in what do you place your hope when the bottom falls out?"

The first actor portrayed an alcoholic named Carlton, who had placed his hope in a sponsor. His sponsor fell off the wagon after ten years. Carlton's hope was lost and he fell off too, losing his family to drinking.

Up next was an engineer who had placed all his trust in his degrees: BA, MA, PhD, BMW and MTA. The audience cackled. When he was laid off, his wife, who had no degrees, found a job without much effort. Disillusioned, he watched TV all day and complained that the men at work were looking at his wife with interest. Someone in the crowd hollered for him to quit being jealous of his wife, turn off the TV and look for a job. Comments from the audience were sometimes comical, sometimes thought-provoking. Spectators booed and hissed a man who kept making negative comments.

During a "commercial break," there was an ad for SlimFast. A young man was padded and dressed to look like an overweight woman. They even borrowed my hat to complete his outfit. He played the "before;" a very skinny girl played the "after." The audience went to pieces.

Playing the part of an anorexic, a young girl shared that, since her parents divorced, she stayed in her room, starving herself and avoiding her friends. A young man in the audience offered her his friendship. He spoke in earnest, as if he had forgotten it was only a play. My nephew, Jamal, told me that the young man really had a crush on the girl.

"Put your hands together and welcome my next guest, coming all the way from California! Give a round of applause to my sister, Joy!"

A young man escorted me to the stage. Faith introduced me, explaining that I had graciously agreed to talk about my journey through some recent life-changing traumas. I discussed the divorce, the legal battle, my mother's death, and the cancer diagnosis. I shared several poems that expressed my decision to trust God no matter what.

Carlton, the alcoholic, asked me why I hadn't given up with all the bad things that kept happening. I replied that I had learned to recognize small blessings. As those added up, I realized that, if a big God could care about the little things in my life, then surely I could trust Him with the big things. I could find God in the difficult times, if I look for Him, remembering that sunshine will follow the rain. My closing poem was "God Will Work It All Out."

When I returned to my table, a woman rushed over to me in tears. She had thought I was acting too, then realized my story was true. Her sister was going through a separation and had been recently diagnosed with bilateral breast and brain cancer. She thought the poem "Breast Pain" could help her sister. I was flabbergasted! I reached for the poem, but she stopped me.

"What I really want is for you to talk to her. I believe she is not telling us everything because she doesn't want to scare the family. She is not in a support group, so I think you could help her because you are going through it too." We exchanged phone numbers.

"Wow!" I thought. "Is this why God brought me to Boston this weekend?"

I was greeted by a friend of my mother whose husband had died a week before Mama. She had been grieving deeply and my poems encouraged her. While thanking me, she pressed some cash into my hand. "Keep up the good work! I will be praying for you." Many people registered their gratitude for my honest sharing, telling me how much I had blessed them. I was equally blessed by their generous spirits.

The music seemed especially tailor-made for me. One song, "He'll Do It Again" (by Shirley Caesar), talked about how God rescued Daniel from the lion's den and the three Hebrew boys from the fiery furnace. He did it for them and He'll do it again for me. My faith was strengthened and my heart encouraged, as I contemplated the fiery furnace of chemotherapy and radiation that awaited me. God didn't keep the Hebrew boys from being thrown in the fire, but He was in it with them.

The service on Sunday morning was another special blessing. I had goose bumps as the trio again sang my song. The worship celebration was especially joyous and uplifting. God was filling up the tank for my new journey.

That evening, as Faith and I talked, my scalp started itching. As I scratched, my hair began to shed.

Faith and Jamal said goodbye and left for work and school on Monday morning. Daddy stopped by a West Indian Market, where I purchased some treats for Avizi and Agalia. We then visited Mama's grave. I didn't feel any particular emotions, but asked Daddy whether he thought Mama could see what I was going through. He didn't think so. He said the Bible doesn't tell us that. All the same, I wondered.

"Where will I be buried when my time comes?" I asked him.

"In California, of course!" he replied, missing the implication of my question.

I was back home when my helper, Clarissa, judiciously suggested, "You have bald patches all over your head. You may as well take it all off." Bending over the bathroom sink, I brushed my hands across my head. What remained of my hair fell into the sink like dead leaves falling from a plant. Yes, that red devil had done its job and my head was now as bald as a baby's bottom.

185

# FOR EVERYTHING THERE'S A SEASON

We may not know the reason
For all of life's suffering and pain,
But we know everything has its season,
So the sunshine will follow the rain.
There are even times when the sun shines
While the rain is still pouring down,
Those moments of grace God sends us,
Reminders that He's still around.

So when adversity's fire is burning,
Expect a cooling breeze.
Know that God is right in it with you
As He moves your growth to achieve.
Embrace His tender compassion,
But yield to His discipline too,
For the Father loves each of His children
And knows best how to nurture you.

When life's pruning is painful,
Don't let bitterness enter your soul,
For when pruning is done you'll be better,
Your heart and your spirit whole.
So if this is your season for weeping,
Know your tears will end with the night,
For joy will come in the morning
When faith gives way to sight.

"There is a time for everything…a time to plant and a time to uproot…a time to tear down and a time to build, a time to weep and a time to laugh, a time to mourn and a time to dance…"
Ecclesiastes 3:1-4

# RED DEVIL

On May 13<sup>th</sup>, I awoke with a feeling of dread. Taking a few deep breaths to calm my jittery nerves, I quietly sang, "What have I to dread, what have I to fear, leaning on the everlasting arms? I have blessed peace with my Lord so near, leaning on the everlasting arms" (E. A. Hoffman).

It was time for my second dose of chemo and I was experiencing anticipatory nausea. Despite my apprehension, I knew that many people were specifically praying for me that morning. I assured Fanny that it wouldn't take more than 15 to 20 minutes. She needed to be back home for her guests, who were arriving from Hawaii that day.

"I had to clean the bathroom again. My cat vomited and had diarrhea. She does that every time we change her diet."

"Are you sure your cat isn't taking chemo? Maybe I will come home with you. Then you can clean up after both of us."

The doctor assured me that my blood count, taken the previous day, was normal. He could proceed with the treatment.

"I'm giving you an antinausea drug called Decadron," the doctor informed me as he prepared his paraphernalia. I winced as he pushed the needle through my skin and into the catheter. It was the only pain I felt during the procedure.

"You will feel a tingling throughout your body, especially in the groin area. Most of my patients say it is very unpleasant."

"Aren't you going to give me Kytril again?"

"Yes, I'm giving you both. Are you feeling the tingling yet?" Several queries later, I still wasn't tingling.

"You're a tough lady," he responded in surprise. I was sitting on the edge of the table with the back raised for support, not the most comfortable position. An IV tube dangled from a pole, and the other end was attached to the needle in my catheter. He was adding Adriamycin, the so-called "red devil."

"Be sure to tell me if it burns, because if it does, we are in big trouble."

"What would you do if it does burn?"

"We would have to stop immediately. You could get an ulcer bad enough to need a skin graft."

"Yikes!" I thought. Suddenly, the tingling was in my head, face and neck. I also had a metallic taste in my mouth. "It's happening! I'm starting to tingle!"

Emptying the last of three vials of Adriamycin (150 mg), the doctor warned me, "Try not to get pregnant. This drug is very toxic and the baby would be born deformed."

"Not a chance," I laughed. "Only one virgin birth in history."

The next treatment was set for June 5th. My son's eighth grade graduation would be June 12th. I hoped I would have enough time to recover. On the way home, we stopped at Mervyn's to exchange a baseball hat for a fancy straw hat to complement the outfit I planned to wear. Though bald, I was having fun with hats and appreciated not having to pay a hairdresser for the next year.

At about five o'clock, the nausea set in. A friend brought dinner from El Pollo Loco. One whiff of the chicken told me I wouldn't be eating. The children were oblivious to my suffering as they chomped down. I vomited several times that night and finally sank into an exhausted sleep.

For several days, I was in agony. This was only the second of 12 treatments. How would I do it? I wanted to cry but was afraid it would only make me sicker, so I restrained myself. Nothing tasted good and there was a burning sensation in my esophagus and stomach. I tried an antacid, but threw that up along with the antinausea pill.

"Don't think about the ten more treatments," a friend encouraged. "That will overwhelm you. It's like standing at the bottom of a high mountain you are about to climb. You don't think you can ever reach the top, and you don't even want to start. Try to focus on one treatment at a time, and getting through that." She was right.

# MISSING MAMA

It was approximately five months after my mastectomy. I had another dream about Mama. In this dream, I found myself in Boston, attending a memorial service held in her honor. I was late and very agitated, as I slipped into a pew near the back. Even at the funeral, I hadn't been that upset. Life's shocks had so sedated me, I had sung a solo during the service with great composure.

In the dream, Faith, also distraught, approached me. "Did Daddy tell you we have some mementos of Mama on display in the back?"

"No!" I snapped, becoming even more enraged. All I saw in the back was an empty casket. At the sight of it, I whirled around, grabbed hold of the pew in front of me and shook with grief. Throwing my arms in the air, I screamed with everything in me, "God, I'm angry!" I awoke, heard myself screaming, and wept with unrestrained anguish.

"Mama, Mama! Are you in pain?" my daughter called from her room.

"I just dreamed about Mama." I sobbed. It was the first time I had really been able to grieve for her. The sorrow was overwhelming.

A few days later, I discussed this dream and the previous one with my support group. I was experiencing horrible side effects from my second chemo treatment. Some group members mentioned their mothers being there for them. That made me miss mine even more. I missed her when I went to court and I missed her when chemo made me sick. She would have been in the kitchen feeding the children and keeping them out of my hair. What hair? I was already bald!

"Dreams are often symbolic," explained the group facilitator. "Just think. What's in your chest? Your heart, which is symbolic of love, caring and compassion. And what was flowing from her heart? Perhaps the blood represented the fact that she does care about what you are going through. Maybe your mother does know, and the dream was her way of letting you know that she cares."

I nodded my head in appreciation. I supposed I would never know for certain on this side, but it sure was comforting to think so.

# SNAPSHOTS OF MAMA

Born in 1917, Ivy Lucilda became a committed follower of Jesus in her early 20's, and married Claudius James at age 30. Seven robust children, of whom I'm the eldest, were eventually added to their union. Mama's grandfather, a Scottish Caucasian, married her grandmother, a Jamaican of mixed descent. Both my mother and grandmother were of fair complexion. Relatives who had bought the White lie that Black meant "less than" objected to my parents' union on the basis that Daddy was "too black and too poor." Nevertheless, Ivy and Claudius defied their criticism and stayed the course.

A woman rich in faith, Ivy was committed to right living. As children, we did not know we were poor. Mama instilled in us a sense of gratitude for the smallest blessing. She impressed us with the importance of honesty and integrity by example, strong reprimands and whippings. Her admonitions were often delivered in rhyme: "It is a sin to steal a pin, much more a greater thing;" and "Speak the truth and speak it ever, cost it what it will; he who hides the wrong he does, does the wrong thing still." "Willful waste brings woeful want" reminded us not to trivialize our blessings.

Exasperated by our misbehavior, Mama would raise eyes and hand to Heaven crying, "Jesus, Savior, pilot me!" If your name followed, you were in trouble! I would have picked Mama's whipping over her severe lectures any day. With her finger in your face, she would quote from the King James Bible: "He that stiffeneth his neck shall be suddenly cut off, and that, without remedy (Proverbs 29:1);" or, "It is a fearful thing to fall into the hands of a living God (Hebrews 10:31)." To the child who bristled at her rebuke, she would declare, "...He that hateth reproof is brutish (Proverbs 12:1)." We knew not to ignore Mama when she warned, "Come straight home from school today; I had a bad dream last night."

In the era of outdoor plumbing, chamber pots, coal and kerosene stoves, and cooking everything from scratch, Mama's labor was hard. She often remarked, "You won't finish housework, but it will finish you." The Queen of Clean, Mama believed that "cleanliness is next to godliness." She scrubbed and disinfected, inside and out, even boiled bed linens and undergarments. Her attempt to protect her brood from jiggers, ringworm and easily transmitted diseases sometimes failed.

Mama and I contracted mumps at the same time. I retain the vivid image of our swollen faces swaddled in bay rum-soaked nappies (baby diapers) that were knotted on top of our heads. Mama could concoct herbal remedies for most ailments, so we rarely saw a doctor. Her children were regularly dosed with castor oil followed by Epsom salts or Senna tea to eliminate parasites. Irregularity was addressed with brown soap enemas. We washed our hands with carbolic soap and Dettol was poured into our bath water.

My parents' efforts to minimize negative influences weren't always successful, though we changed residences a few times. However, Mama, not a fatalist, would say, "Do you notice the lily? It grows in mud but always comes out white." She taught us that dependence on God and commitment to His standards were the keys to true success. Mama felt that education, though essential, was not the most important thing because "there are a lot of educated fools in the world." If someone called her foolish for believing in Jesus, she would respond, "I am a fool for Christ! Whose fool are you?"

Believing that "prayer changes things," Mama committed each of her children to God while we were still in her womb. Many were the stories of God's providential interventions when Mama prayed. Sometimes she petitioned Him for the next meal. The answer often arrived while she was still on her knees. Both parents prayed us through good times and bad, Mama encouraging, "Lean hard on God's promises; you can't break them."

Ivy, called Mama by many, also implored Heaven for those she considered her spiritual children. Her petitions blanketed "those on land, sea, and in the air." Her prayerful intervention kept a young woman from aborting her baby. The new mother expressed her gratitude at Mama's memorial service.

In Ivy's house, hearth and heart were open to anyone with a need. A cousin often ran with her baby to that "city of refuge" to escape her abusive husband. A friend who lived in the suburbs sometimes passed through on her way home from work. She recalls, "Mrs. Walker always had a little something to hold me till I got home to cook for my family."

Mama had an uncanny way of discerning people's needs. After cooking a pot of soup, she would dash off to take some for "Mrs. Whoever," and would return with incredible stories of rescue: An elderly woman without heat in the cold of winter, or a victim of domestic violence with a broken ankle and no heat or food. Mama and her soup were always "God-sent."

I learned creative cooking from Mama, who never owned a cookbook. She could produce a scrumptious dish from pinches of this, a dab of that, and a handful of the other. When there was more month than money, or less food than mouths to feed, Mama would rustle up a meal from not so popular ingredients, then grin mischievously as we licked our chops and begged for more.

Practical wisdom was Ivy's forte, though she only had a sixth grade education. When my siblings and I squabbled over a Paradise Plum, Mama would crush the candy and make us share the crumbs. Her conversation with another adult was often interrupted by bickering children. Ivy would throw handfuls of corn kernels in the yard, then send the kids to retrieve them. As they merrily scrambled off to see who would find the most, she would continue her conversation in peace.

We learned many songs of faith from Mama; some still help me fight life's battles, such as, "Whisper a prayer in the morning…To keep your heart in tune." When I was worried, she sang, "Why worry when you can pray…? Ivy often bolstered our faith with the song, "Cheer up ye saints of God, there's nothing to worry about… remember Jesus never fails…You'll be sorry you worried at all tomorrow morning" (anonymous). Mama was often heard pouring out her heart to God in anguished sobs. Then, she would rise from her knees and saunter down the hall with a smiling, tear-stained face, singing, "The hotter the battle, the sweeter the victory!"

Even from her bed of affliction, Mama reminded us to "Brighten up your pathway with a song." I had the invaluable and unforgettable privilege of singing some of those songs back to Mama just a few weeks before she left for Heaven. Now she's singing with the angels and her voice will forever echo in my memory.

"Only one life, twill soon be past,
Only what's done for Christ will last."—Charles Studd

## TAKING THE BULL BY THE HORNS

Agalia had been unhappy and stressed all year. She kept badgering me about my promise to move her to our church school as soon as Avizi graduated. That promise had been made before my cancer diagnosis. I wasn't so sure now. The child was devastated. One day, she complained that her teacher had embarrassed her in front of the class about her handwriting, and some students had tormented her. I called the principal at our church school.

"I promised to transfer her, but that was before life threw me a curve ball. Now I am dealing with cancer and chemotherapy. I'm afraid to bite off more than I can chew. I need to bounce this off someone wise. The decision is hard for me as a single mom. Do you think I am being foolhardy for even considering it?"

"Frankly, if you have a child that age who really wants to be in a Christian school, you should do it if at all possible." The principal reminded me of the church membership discount and available scholarships. "We're testing and there is still room in the sixth grade. Trust God with the finances. Go ahead and apply. Your daughter needs to be in a supportive environment. She will certainly have that here. Our staff has been praying for you regularly."

The following day, the school secretary assured me, "You had her tested last year. We'll arrange to test her again, but you don't have to pay for it. We want to have you here. We'll support you and will be praying for you." Her compassion moved me to tears. Agalia was ecstatic!

"Mom, I know this will be a harder school, but that is what I need; I need to be challenged."

A few weeks later, she came home very agitated. Her teacher asked if anyone was not returning the next year. Agalia disclosed that she would be transferring to a private school. According to her, the teacher scowled and looked at her weird. At recess, some students teased her, saying she would flunk and have to come back.

That afternoon, the class was given a creative writing assignment. Agalia unleashed her fury in her story: Two gigantic spiders attacked everyone at the school, creating widespread chaos. I could hear her anger as she read it to me. Concerned about retaliation, I wrote the teacher a letter.

On receiving it, she allegedly took my daughter outside, so enraged that the letter shook in her hand. She accused my child of telling me "all lies," and called my letter to her "all lies;" claimed I was blaming her for my illness. I was livid!

"Mom, she was so mad and I was so scared that I just kept my mouth shut and prayed in my heart that God would make her stop."

"This time I am writing a letter to the principal," I declared, my blood hot. A conference was scheduled for the week after my third chemo treatment.

The principal questioned Agalia, "You said she scowled and looked at you weird. How can you interpret a look?"

"I am visually impaired, but my daughter is not," I intervened.

"Yes, but a scowl could have meant any number of things. Your daughter is a very bright girl. At least we helped identify that for you this year." (What made her think I didn't know that?) She turned to the teacher, "If I had heard she wasn't coming back, I would have had a look of disappointment or surprise, wouldn't you?"

I was thinking, but didn't say, "There's a big difference between a look of surprise and disappointment and a nasty scowl. Wouldn't a 'very bright girl' know the difference?"

"I did not scowl! All kinds of accusations have come at me all year," whined the teacher.

"We had a conference at the beginning of the year, right here," I reminded her. "I have not come to you with any other complaint until now." One of the reasons for the previous conference was to address the teacher's yelling at Agalia about her handwriting. She went on about how much she had tried all year to help her, with no improvement. Agalia then whipped out her story and handed it to the principal.

"I remember looking at her handwriting at the beginning of the year, and I definitely see improvement here," the principal (not the teacher) admitted. I pointed out that it had already been established that this was an area of weakness for my child. Yelling at her in front of the class was embarrassing, discouraging, and certainly not the way to help her.

"I never yell!" yelled the teacher, her dander up.

Unruffled, Agalia retorted, "You yell every single day! Some of the kids asked me what this conference was about, and I told them. They are willing to come in here and say that she does yell at me." This was directed to the principal. It was ignored, of course.

"This girl came to school with an attitude," the teacher countered. "She is a bright child, and delightful, but it was her first day in school. She had trouble with her handwriting because she was homeschooled. It's what she wasn't taught." I think it's clear who had the attitude.

"What do you know about what she was or wasn't taught? Have all your students always caught everything you taught, and if so, why aren't you being lauded in the media as Teacher of the Year?" That is what I was thinking, but said instead, "The purpose of this conference is to deal with the fact that I addressed a letter to you, the teacher, in which I appealed to your sensitivity toward my daughter. Your response was most unprofessional! Rather than contacting me via writing or telephone, you did the very thing I asked you not to do, traumatize the child again. You flew into a rage, accused her of lying, and told her I was blaming you for my illness." I turned to the principal. "Why would I blame her for my illness? Why would I ascribe such power to her? I scarcely know her!"

"I was not angry when I spoke to her. I simply told her that the things she had told you weren't true."

Agalia replied with confidence, "You were so angry that your hands shook with the letter!" She told me later that the teacher turned red at that juncture. That woman was not about to own up to anything.

"Well, it's her word against mine! You know you can't always believe a child," was her cowardly defense.

"And you can't always believe an adult," I should have said. I retorted dryly instead, "I know when to believe mine, and I do not believe you." I repeated it for emphasis. At this point, the principal, wisely summing up the situation, suggested that Agalia spend the remaining days of the semester with the other fifth grade teacher. As we wrapped things up, the principal cordially shook my hand and wished me the best. The teacher sat glumly, her hands in her lap. I extended mine, calling her name.

"When you sent Agalia to talk with your friend who had a mastectomy, I thought it a very kind gesture, and I told her so. I am here to be my daughter's advocate in this specific issue. Thank you. Goodbye." She reluctantly shook my hand.

I addressed Agalia directly: "I hope you learned something from this. If someone wrongs you, do not be afraid to confront them; if you are in the right, stand tall, look them in the eye and respectfully speak the truth. Always maintain your dignity and don't allow yourself to be bullied by anyone. Never lower yourself to the level of your opponent. There are many who will question your intelligence or disregard your abilities; some will trivialize you because you are a girl, or belittle you because of the color of your skin. Don't let them cause you to lose faith in yourself. Remember, it is God who establishes your value, not misdirected people."

My child was very proud of herself for acting "like an adult," but was somewhat apprehensive about going to school the next day. The two teachers were friends, and she wasn't sure what to expect. I sang to her the song from *The King and I*. "Whenever I feel afraid, I hold my head erect and whistle a happy tune, so no one will suspect I'm afraid." The next morning, I smiled as I heard her singing it on the way out. In spite of her misgivings, Agalia made the honor roll again, and the other teacher gave her a certificate of appreciation for perseverance.

I was in fighting mode. I was standing up to cancer and ready for any other challenge. Bring it!

# PATIENT ACTIVISM

"Three strikes, he's out!"

My first chemo treatment made me very sick. The oncologist knew his medicine but not his patient. He made no attempt to understand the emotional intensity of my experience.

I was derailed by the extreme side effects of Decadron, the antinausea medication. I thought I was losing my mind. The oncologist said it was all in my head and that I needed a psychiatrist. On my next visit, I voiced the same complaint. This time he acknowledged it was caused by the medicine. When he denied having said the symptoms were in my head, I found that quite disconcerting. If I hadn't had my friend Rosie with me on each visit, I might have bought the lie, but I had a witness.

A member of my support group had used this drug. She said I wasn't crazy. She had been a Decadron junkie. The information gave me more courage to confront the doctor. When I declined the drug, he told me how sick I would be. I wondered how I would survive 12 chemo treatments.

The best *encouragement* my oncologist could offer was that two percent of people receiving chemo don't really need it and are being poisoned. Should that have inspired me to complete the course? After my fourth treatment, he suspended chemo to start radiation. I was not going back to him!

The radiation oncologist was very upset. "I have to live with my conscience. I will not do anything to jeopardize your chances of recovery." She strongly suggested I return to the other doctor for my fifth chemo treatment. It had already been delayed in the transition. She didn't understand why he had interrupted chemo to start radiation. Her recommendation for a mastectomy had been correct, so I trusted her. I was traumatized by the whole affair.

Before taking the fifth chemo treatment, I requested Zofran, an antinausea drug recommended by members of my support group. The doctor refused my request, saying it was too expensive. This doctor was clearly not going to be my advocate. I called my HMO and found that Zofran was on the list of approved drugs. I demanded it and had no nausea or vomiting for five days. Exhilarated, I wrote "Antinausea Cheer," then vomited the following day. Maybe I was too excited.

Three strikes and he was out. It was my ball game, not his. I put the wheels in motion and dismissed that doctor. Fighting cancer has definitely taught me the importance of being my own advocate. I learned to trust my God-given intuition. Medicine is an art and doctors are not little gods, though they wield a great deal of power. Becoming actively involved in my treatment equipped me to make informed decisions with confidence. Belonging to a support group made the gathering of information much easier. It gave me the courage to demand what I needed.


## *ANTINAUSEA CHEER*

Hurrah for Zofran! Hurrah for Zofran!
I can eat, don't have to reach for my vomitorium.
I can smell and taste and slurp, even make a healthy burp.
I no longer have to lurch in regurgitation.
Hurrah for Zofran!


## *IT'S MY BALL GAME*
(Tune: "Take Me Out to the Ball Game")

My doctor did not understand me,
He did not even try.
He treated me just like a guinea pig.
Now I may be fat but I'm nobody's pig!

I'm a woman with real emotions,
Traumatized, hurting and scared,
But Doc just pushed the drugs as if it were
His own ball game.

I asked my doctor for Zofran.
He wouldn't give it to me.
Instead, he injected some Decadron
Which made me flip, I knew something was wrong,
But would you believe what he told me?
He said, "It's all in your head
And I think that you need a shrink."
And I thought, "That stinks!"

I got rid of my doctor.
He was not good for me.
I almost stopped chemo because of him.
What he said and did made the future look grim,
So one day, I called up my HMO
And said, "I need someone new!"
For it's 1-2-3 strikes, he's out!
'Cause it's my ball game!

The moral of the story is:
Be patient-active always.
You must pay attention to what you feel,
Your personal power will help you get healed.
So go take charge of your health care,
You pay that doctor big bucks.
Now please be polite but don't be too nice,
'Cause it's your ball game!

# NEW DOCTOR, NEW HOPE

"You weigh 200 lbs.?" queried the nurse as she peered at the scale. "You sure don't look it."

"Ah, well!" I sighed. "I heard that weight loss was one of the side effects of chemo and was hoping it would be a benefit for me, but it sure isn't happening."

"Don't even think about it! That's the least of your priorities. Right now you just want to get well."

I handed her the pathology slides and chemo records from the former oncologist. He had not said a word regarding his dismissal. I had not been inclined to waste my limited energy to give him a piece of my mind, as some had suggested. I needed all of it for myself.

When we were ushered into the office of Dr. Bonito, a medical oncologist at Breast Cancer Clinic, the warmth of her greeting impressed me immediately. I felt really good about taking charge of my life in this way. Dr. Bonito spent time getting to know me. She studied my records, then listened attentively as I explained my reason for the transfer.

I told her of my frightening mood swings after using Decadron, and how the other doctor had said it was all in my head. She informed me that a side effect of that drug was steroidal psychosis. I shuddered, then sighed with relief, "Thank God I got rid of that doctor!"

Convinced that Mama's demise was hastened by drugs, I would not use any medication that wasn't absolutely necessary. Without chemotherapy, I knew the cancer could metastasize. Still I had wanted to quit.

Dr. Bonito explained that the former oncologist had based his treatment protocol on an old study. It mandated 12 treatments: four with the drug Adriamycin and eight with a combination of Methotrexate, 5FU and Cytoxan. A more recent study proved that 12 treatments were no more effective than eight. I had been looking at seven more, but now there would be just three.

"Only three more!" I gasped with delight. At last, there was a light at the end of the tunnel and it wasn't a train. My intuitive self had been warning me all along. No wonder I had wanted to quit. What might have happened had I not trusted my intuition? Three more seemed so much better than seven!

Dr. Bonito questioned me about my personal history, demonstrating her interest in me as a person, and not just as a patient. She scribbled notes while quizzing me about my siblings' names, ages and medical history. She also urged me to tell my sisters to get their mammograms done regularly. They were at risk for breast cancer, as was my daughter. My friend, Chris, mentioned that I was a poet. The doctor showed interest, so I shared "Breast Pain" from memory. She was touched and expressed a desire to hear more.

A new, meaningful relationship was formed in one visit, something that hadn't happened in ten visits with the previous oncologist. After a thorough exam, I went home knowing that Cancer Clinic was the place for me. I looked forward to having my follow-up done in a caring environment. When Dr. Bonito called to schedule the next chemo treatment, she was so upbeat! I beamed with relief. I knew my HMO would authorize the change. After all, they were being saved the cost of four unnecessary treatments.

## *JOURNEY OF FAITH*

When circumstances hurl themselves
Against my trembling soul,
My charged emotions ride the waves
Up and down, around and around,
Reaching out with arms of faith
To the Orchestrator of the crashing sounds.
I know He has a plan I cannot see.
Anxiously I search for Him
And find Him watching me.
When I'm swept beneath the waves,
He gently lifts me up,
And carries me safely in His arms,
For He is strong!

Then when He puts me down again,
I can with strength go on.
When, like Peter, I begin to falter,
His voice says calmly, "Come."
Then with my gaze on Him,
I move with measured steps
Through torrents of tears
And wild relentless winds
Of unanswered questions.
Deliberately I push aside
Fears that loom malevolent,
Climbing through barriers of despair
To find my feet on higher ground
Where I've not walked before.
When blinded by life's present pain,
I won't give in to fears I feel.
But look to God with eyes of faith.
I know His love is real!

# PART 10. REACHING OUT

## SAY IT NOW

We often wait till someone's gone
To say how much she's meant to us,
Yet all of us have moments when
We doubt our true significance
And need strong reassurance
That our being has helped light the way
For others in their struggles.
So take the time to bring to mind
The people who've inspired you,
Then let them know right now, today,
Your deep appreciation.
We may not always realize
How some kind word
That's timely spoken
May boost the wavering spirit
Of one we have considered strong
Who now may need the encouragement
Derived from a sincere compliment.


## SAYING GOODBYE

After a support group meeting, I laid in bed sleepless and painfully aware of the suffering represented in the group. "Lord," I prayed fervently, "I know you have me in this group for a reason. How can I help? What can I give?"

I thought of Mary, who had been fighting metastatic breast cancer since 1993. She had tried everything: bone marrow stem cell rescue, chemotherapy and radiation. The cancer was in her bones after only a brief remission. Mary was heavily medicated and receiving blood transfusions. I watched her steady decline since first joining the group in March. It was now September. Mary was in her late 50's. Her parents, in their 80's, had moved into her apartment to help care for her. Mary was a conscientious worker and quitting her job was hard.

We were inspired as we watched Mary move through the various stages of preparation for dying. She deliberated giving prized possessions to loved ones. She did not want items with sentimental value just carted off from a yard sale by some stranger unaware of their significance. Setting her financial and family affairs in order was important to her, yet she hoped her suffering wouldn't be too long.

I wanted to reach out to Mary, but wasn't sure how. What could one give a person who was dying? So often we wait till we have lost someone to vocalize their value to us. It had been such a blessing to celebrate my parents' 48th anniversary shortly before Mama died. Pondering the importance of such a tribute, I decided to write Mary a poem. It would encourage her and could be left for her loved ones.

When I called to make sure Mary would attend the meeting, she sounded groggy and weak. The medication made her very sleepy. She wasn't sure she could stay awake for two hours. I insisted she needed to be there. We missed her and I had something special for her. She instantly perked up, admitting she missed the group too. Her parents, Mal and Merle, would bring her for part of the time.

I was not prepared for the feeble woman escorted into the room by her elderly parents. That she had lost a considerable amount of weight was evident, even to my impaired vision. Unlike the other group members, I was spared the pain of viewing the more pronounced signs of her decline. My stomach tightened. I pulled myself together in order to share the poem. It had been almost a year since Mama died. Seeing Mary brought back memories. Mama also had been reduced to bones.

Mary's voice was weak as she explained the infusion pump which gave her doses of pain medication intermittently. She was simply managing the pain and waiting for the end. Her voice trailed away frequently as she spoke. It must have taken a supreme effort for her to come to the meeting.

"I don't see how anyone can live on drugs for recreation," Mary mused. The box of Kleenex was passed around as I read the poem. A few tears trickled down my cheek, but I was too numb to cry like the others. When I handed Mary her printed copy, she remarked with her usual wit, "I can definitely read this copy better than I can read your Braille." Everyone tittered through their tears. She said no one had ever written her a poem. She would leave it for her son. The other group members shared how Mary had been an inspiration in her struggles.

Mary became very drowsy. We all hugged and caressed her, saying our goodbyes. After she left the room, group members continued crying and sharing. Our group leader remarked that, of all the groups she had facilitated, ours was the first one that had ever said goodbye like this.

"How could you read the poem without falling apart?" queried Diana, as she wiped her nose. I shared how close to home this experience was. I recalled singing at Mama's funeral, too numb to feel the deep pain that had lodged in my heart.

I had also written a poem for Bobs, a former child actor and Methodist minister. He played the role of Pee Wee in the movie "Boy's Town." Deeply depressed and lonely, he wished death would come soon. His poem was titled "Don't Be Afraid of Living." He thanked me for the love with which I wrote it and promised to read it many times. We never saw Bobs again.

Later that night, I clutched my stomach in pain, feeling profound sadness and a sense of futility. The following day, I was a basket case. The numbness had gone and the delayed reaction had come. I cried unhindered, grieving for my mother, for Mary, for Bobs, for myself and for all cancer sufferers. I talked to Janet, who had been in the meeting the previous evening. She was attentive and empathetic as I unloaded.

The harsh reality of human suffering brings to mind the Lord Jesus hanging on the cross. His was a substitutionary death. The full weight of human misery fell on Him. He died and was resurrected, bringing us hope for a better life after our sorrows here are over. Some people ask why a loving God allows suffering. They fail to see that it was such a loving God who sent His Son into the midst of the desolation to show us a way through it and back to Himself.

Pain is a reality because we live in a broken, sinful world; however, we need not endure it without purpose. If we embrace God's intervention through the death and resurrection of Jesus; if we accept the hope God offers us through an intimate relationship with Himself—then even from the depths of anguish, our spirits can rejoice in the promise of eternity without sickness or crying or pain. Jesus said He is preparing a place of joy and peace and will someday take me there. I pray that my journey will inspire someone to seek refuge and strength in God (Psalm 46:1).

Mary died on October 17th, 1997, three weeks after our last meeting.

## SISTERS IN SUFFERING

God let us step into each other's lives
For one short act: "Sisters in Suffering."
Though which of us will exit first
Is still the Playwright's secret.
But as I watch,
The style and grace with which you move
Towards the final ending
Fill me with wonder and resolve
To show such poise at my departing.
I pray I'll be as fortunate as you,
With time to fix unfinished business,
Bequeathing love's last gifts to those held dear,
Surrendering them to life and to God's care.
I hope I'll be a mirror of Christ's peace,
Blessed memory for those bereaved to keep;
And when the curtain falls upon life's stage,
May both our souls awake on Heaven's side,
Where Jesus will be our Eternal Guide.

Dedicated to Mary

# DON'T BE AFRAID OF LIVING

Your tears of loneliness touch my heart
And I cried too,
For I have known such grief:
The realization that I'd falsely hoped
In love that really wasn't there;
The feeling I could not outswim
Waves of rejection threatening to engulf me;
The rain of pain that soaked my spirit;
The wish for death to lull me
Into deep forgetful sleep.

The God you've served with all your heart
Now stands near with tearful eyes,
His fingers beckoning you to come
Curl up in His almighty arms.
Smothering your sorrows in His love,
He'll hold you there till all your tears are shed.
I do not think He wants you dead
Before you've come to understand
How He can fill the empty spaces,
Sending His love through many faces,
Infusing life with indescribable joy
That triumphs over pain.

So grieve your loss, then let it go,
Stretch out your arms to friends who'll give
To you some of the love you've given.
Don't be afraid of living.

Dedicated to Robert B. "Bobs" Watson, 1930-1999

# *PUT WHAT LITTLE FAITH YOU HAVE IN HIM*

When problems box you in on every side,
When fears and dangers make you want to hide,
Small as a grain of mustard seed
Is all the faith you need
To see the hand of God upon your life.
Just be patient and wait for Him to move
And as you wait, to you His love He'll prove.

Refrain:
He'll give you streams in the desert to water your soul,
He'll send you manna from Heaven to make you whole,
You will find wealth in the waiting for God's in control,
Just put what little faith you have in Him.

When you have been betrayed by one you love,
Just bring your broken heart to God above.
He is the one who made it,
So believe that He can mend it,
And wait till He again restores your joy.
You can trust Him for He was once betrayed;
As you trust Him, your night He'll turn to day. (Refrain)

When pain and sickness tear your body down,
When boulders crush your dreams and hope lays torn,
Just turn your tear-filled eyes,
He's right there as you cry,
And with His bottle catches every tear.
Let Him hold you as you walk through the rain,
Let Him love you, however deep the pain. (Refrain)

"...be strong, do not fear; your God will come...Then will the lame leap for joy...Water will gush forth in the wilderness and streams in the desert...The burning sand will become a pool, the thirsty ground bubbling springs." Isaiah 35:4-7

## DON'T WEEP FOR ME AS IF I'M LOST

Yes, I suffered much and long
While my body-temple weakened,
But the Lord stayed close to me
And my spirit daily strengthened.

As my house of clay was falling
And I quickly slipped away,
I could hear my Savior calling;
This is what I heard Him say:

"Precious daughter, come up higher!
Come into your rest divine!
You have fought the fight with honor!
Now my child, you are all mine!

Where I am there's joy eternal,
For the sting of death is past,
No more fear nor pain nor peril
Will ever again invade your heart.

Here no suffering ever enters,
No more tears and no more night,
Perfect peace here reigns, triumphant,
I Am The King! I Am The Light!"

Don't weep for me as if I'm lost,
For I'm in the arms of Jesus.
Free at last from all restraints
I'm worshipping my Savior.

Eyes have not seen, nor ears heard
The welcome He prepared for me,
A welcome He will give to any
Who to Him will bow the knee.

Open up your heart to Jesus,
Come taste and see that God is good!
Greater love no one can show
Than Christ did when He shed His blood for you!

Dedicated to Linda Rueles, who died on August 19th, 1998, after battling ovarian cancer. Linda had asked me to write a poem about Heaven. This was written four days after her death.


## FLOWER IN GOD'S HANDS

Precious, though fragile,
Held in God's hands with great care
Because He chose you.
Rare perfume escapes
As God's sovereign hands squeeze you
For His own purpose.
Fragrant aroma
Spreads to those who observe you,
Bruised yet beautiful.

Dedicated to Elsie Purnell (1935-2005) & Paula Dinkins (1952-2011)


## THIS IS WHAT I PRAY

The Master Designer created you
With His own purpose and plan.
May your life, however long,
Honor Him and bless your fellow man.

May He, in His mercy, empower you
As you persevere through this test.
May your fight, however tough,
Inspire us to live our very best.

May all the memories that we have shared
Put a smile on your face.
May the times of joy that made us laugh
Comfort you and some measure of pain erase.

May the Great Physician, the God of Hope,
Bring blessings abundant each day.
May His healing hands caress your soul
And make you whole—this is what I pray.

Dedicated to Elizabeth Terry (1962-2007)


## FAITHFUL FRIEND

It was a special moment when
The Lord ordained us to be friends
And chose the proper time and place
When I should meet you face to face.
We've made a bond that's grown more strong
As the years have passed along.
Tears and laughter we have shared
And in my grief you've always cared.

Through all you've been a faithful friend,
So quick a helping hand to lend.
Mercy genuine and true
Is the gift I've seen in you.
Thanks for all you've said and done,
Thanks for many hours of fun,
Thanks for opening heart and home,
Thanks for all the love you've shown!

Dedicated to Gloria and Ruby

## SISTER FRIEND

You often were my counselor
When counsel wise I lacked.
I even trusted you to guard
The deepest secrets of my heart.
We have dreamed and visualized,
Some dreams we've even realized.
You closed neither eye nor ear
To any of my pleas for help,
But stretched out your hand
When I needed a hand to grasp.
Even in my darkest hour,
Your contagious laughter
Or some kind word
Dispelled the gloom,
Making me laugh too.
Though time moves on
And people are forgotten,
Forever and for everything
You are remembered and loved.

Dedicated to my sister, Faith


## YOU'VE MADE A DIFFERENCE

My cup of suffering had overflowed
When God to me His mercy showed.
His heart was moved by my pain and fear,
He knew just how much I could bear.
So keen was He my need to attend,
Into my life He chose to send
Those with His heart, His hands, His feet,
Who would in the trenches with me meet;

Friends who came bringing another cup
With love and empathy filled up,
Holding it gently to my lips
As I their true compassion sipped.
Some prayed for me without reserve,
While others so generously served,
Unmindful of what they'd receive
Save the joy of knowing they could relieve
The burden of another's pain,
By offering a cup in Jesus' Name.
Through your kindness my strength has grown.
Into my darkness, God's light you've shown.
You've made a difference in my sphere
And I'm so grateful that you care! 1998

Dedicated to all my caring friends

# PART 11. MOVING ON

## IS IT REALLY OVER?

By the end of January 1998, after eight rounds of chemotherapy and 36 radiation treatments, I was almost done. My cancer was estrogen-positive, so I was placed on Tamoxifin, an oral medication, for five years. The first chemo had launched me into menopause, deepening my already present depression. Extreme exhaustion prohibited journaling. My entire body ached and lying in bed didn't bring relief. *Chemo brain* short-circuited concentration. Parental responsibilities intensified, as the power struggle with teenagers began.

The group facilitator said it wasn't uncommon for depression to settle in after treatment. Doctor visits were reduced to every three months. I wondered what was happening in my body between visits. During treatment, I had been actively fighting the disease, knowing the cancer cells were being destroyed. Now what? I would have to wait five years for the cancer to be considered in remission. What if it came back?

I continued in group and was terrified each time someone came in with a recurrence. A woman, in remission for 11 years, showed up one evening. The fear was palpable. Can anyone ever be sure it's over? Would I make it to five years? I heard of someone else whose cancer returned after 15 years. It was in her bones, liver and brain. While at The Wellness Community (TWC), I made several friends whom I lost to cancer.

Hoping that life would get better and joy would be restored, I continued my involvement in the support community. I joined the Wellness Connection, a support group for survivors no longer in treatment. I became a survivor-speaker at various events, sharing my journey through poetry. In April of 1998, I was asked to speak at a luncheon sponsored by Kaiser Permanente. Kaiser was making a substantial donation to TWC, which was to be presented at this luncheon.

This was the first time I would speak publicly about my cancer experience. Waiting for a ride, I gathered my thoughts, and within minutes, a poem emerged. I barely had time to write it down (in Braille) and was on my way. At the luncheon, I described my journey and closed with the poem "Each One Helping Each One."

The applause was stunning and exhilarating! I shook hands with many people who were encouraging and supportive. Dr. Kim Ashing was one of the new friends I met that day. She is a cancer research doctor who hails from Trinidad. Our island roots drew us together immediately.

The poem was used in a fund-raising newsletter, the response to which gleaned $5,000 in support for TWC. Although I continued to be involved in various events, cancer was no longer the central focus of my life. My attention was needed more urgently elsewhere.

## *EACH ONE HELPING EACH ONE*

We are all dying, this human race.
We've all been prescribed a time and place.
Living or dying we each blaze a trail.
To those who come after we each tell a tale.
Even my struggles may strengthen another
A few paces behind me, a sister or brother.
The knowledge I gain as I fight for my health,
When shared with others, brings me much wealth.
The sister before me who's losing the fight,
Yet still walks with dignity, gives me insight
Into how I should live 'til it's my time to go.
Each one helping each one is the best way I know
To deal with life's hardships, to soften its blows.
I hope when I'm gone that the trail I have blazed
Will have, for some traveler, a smoother path paved.

## TIME TO SING

I have a song that needs singing
And I want to sing it now!
For too long I have danced
To a tune that's not my own
While my song has been striving to be free.
Its melodious notes I'll let float from my throat
To rise on the wind like a bird that sings
When no one is really listening,
But whose song will wing its way
To a heart that needs cheering,
So I must be sharing my song.
If I don't sing, with my song I will die,
So I must let it fly right now!
It is my time to sing and I won't let a thing
Hold me back or keep me down for I must sing!

"I will sing to the Lord, for he has been good to me." Psalm 13:6

## I WILL LIVE AGAIN

You may snuff out dreams,
But you can't stop my dreaming,
For my soul lives to dream again.
You may spurn my love,
Leave me broken, bruised and bleeding,
Still I know God will heal this pain.
Oh you did break my heart
And the teardrops did flow.
You dragged hope through the gutter,
Yet it doesn't matter now.
I will flush out the pain,
I will live again,
I will climb another mountain,
I will cross another sea.
You can't stop my dreaming
Though you've snuffed out dreams.

## *SONG OF PRAISE*

Lord, Your love overwhelms me,
It is too vast to scan!
The quality of Your mercy humbles me.
Your ways are far above men.
Joy and wonder move my heart
To utter this song of praise.
I cry, but they are tears of joy
As my voice in worship I raise.

For You have removed my transgressions,
Will remember them no more.
What the worm and the canker have eaten,
From Your treasure-house You'll restore.
So long I had lived in quiet fear,
My knowledge of You incomplete,
But now I have found new liberty
And power my sin to defeat.

For the sound of Your voice in my spirit
Has loosened chains from my heart.
Now I know that You really do love me
And for Your use have set me apart.
With all of my heart I praise You
For choosing me as Your own.
May my life's single aim be to serve You
And glorify Your Name alone.

"I will extol the Lord at all times; his praise will always be on my lips. My soul will boast in the Lord; let the afflicted hear and rejoice. Glorify the Lord with me; let us exalt his name together. I sought the Lord, and he answered me; he delivered me from all my fears." Psalm 34:1-4

## BUMP FROM BEHIND

In the fall of 1998, I was advised to get my first colonoscopy. The gastroenterologist informed me that there was a genetic link between breast and colon cancer. The colonoscopy should have taken just 20 minutes, but I had polyps, which had to be removed. Only lightly sedated, I began to moan. I was given more meds. The precancerous polyps were caught just in time. Imagine my consternation at the mention of the "C" word so soon after breast cancer.

My six-month follow-up and several subsequent screenings have been good and are being done every three to five years. If more polyps are found, they can be nipped in the bud. Colon cancer is preventable if screening is done regularly.

The doctor also discovered diverticula, folds or pockets in the lining of the colon which, when inflamed, can cause a very painful condition called diverticulitis. I have had several attacks that sent me to the emergency room in excruciating pain. I was advised to avoid seeds, popcorn and nuts, all very healthy foods. However, with the use of probiotics and an improved diet, I now eat lots of nuts and seeds with no ill effects. My last colonoscopy showed no diverticula or polyps. I will continue to be proactive in fighting off any more surprise attacks from behind.

## MAKING LEMONADE

The first time I had the courage to expose my baldness was to attend a class at the Braille Institute. "That doesn't count," Agalia protested, "they are all blind there." She didn't hear all the whistles and hoots coming from the staff as I arrived, my bald head accented by dangly earrings. An instructor made the comment, "God gave some women hair and the rest He gave beautiful heads." It was an attempt to boost my morale and it did make me chuckle. When I hear women complaining about their hair, I am reminded that a bad hair day is better than a no hair day.

Sometimes, after misplacing my prosthesis, I would run around the house asking, "Have you seen my boob?" My daughter's response always amused me—"Gross!" One Sunday, unable to find my prosthesis, I padded my bra with some old socks and left for church. At a potluck that afternoon, the ladies kept giggling. The men grew curious, which made us laugh even harder. We couldn't tell them what was so funny. They will know now!

Once upon a time, there were two *girls*; one was real, the other was not. The fake one was Caucasian. One day a new *girl* came to town; she was dark-skinned and good-looking. While refitting me with the new prosthesis, my provider suggested, "You can wear the old *girl* every day and keep the new one for dressing up." She was serious.

During water aerobics, I was bent low doing the karate punch when I heard my name. The instructor indicated that I needed to check myself. Looking down, I noticed my prosthesis trying to escape. Grinning, I quickly tucked it in. If it had drifted away, I could have pretended it wasn't mine; wrong color!

"Hello bosom-buddy," my friend Amy greeted me one Sunday morning.

"Hey, what a great name for a club! There are enough of us breast cancer survivors here to start a club. Don't you think?" Amy, 79 years old, had two mastectomies, 27 years apart. She didn't worry about bras or prostheses. She just wore loose blouses or sweaters. As one who had been more than amply endowed, I thought, "If I get cancer in the other breast, God forbid, I will just lop it off, do reconstruction, and triumphantly choose my new breast size."

Checking in at the doctor's office one day, I asked the nurse if I could weigh myself with and without the prosthesis, just to see how heavy it really was. To my chagrin, the thing weighed only three pounds. I expected it to weigh at least ten. During chemotherapy, a nutritionist told me that being overweight is like having money in the bank. I wonder what they call it several years after chemo. In any case, rich as I was, I couldn't expend my pounds in this country. Perhaps I should have gone to London on a shopping spree.

Did you know an artificial boob could double as a weapon of self-defense? Just suppose I was out alone after dark. I could wear the prosthesis outside the bra pocket for easy access. If a deviant should approach (may it never be), intending to mug or something worse, I could instantly whip out my weapon. With the self-confidence and skill gained from several years of strength training, I would, as it were, kill two birds with one boob. I would foil the thug and spoil his mug by covering it with my prosthesis. So profound would be his shock that I could make my getaway, while he tried to decipher what on earth had hit him. Hopefully, I would hit with such force that the imprint on his face would make it easy for the cops to apprehend him.

The next day's headline would read: "Would-be Mugger Upstaged by Breast-wielding Woman," or "Serial Stalker Bamboozled by Black Boob." Sounds great, but there is no guarantee I wouldn't be paralyzed from fear. I don't think pulling out my prosthesis in slow motion would achieve the same end. On second thought, I may not have the chance to slap him with it, but he may be running from sheer fright. Well, that scenario is beyond execution since I no longer wear a prosthesis. I have a new and permanent bosom buddy these days.

Who could have imagined anything funny about cancer? Certainly not me. Well, we're supposed to make lemonade when life gives us lemons, but one person can only drink so much. Enough already!

"A cheerful heart is good medicine, but a crushed spirit dries up the bones." Proverbs 17:22

## *DOOR TO WELLNESS*

When I came to this support group, fear my mind had seized.
I wondered if I would perish from this treacherous disease.
I embraced this new community, my home away from home,
Finding great relief in knowing I was not alone.

When the doors to Wellness opened, hope became my friend,
For mesmerizing stories of victory was the trend.
I harnessed all my powers, prepared for a great fight,
Having comrades in the battle who'd support me in my plight.

I met many people who had already fought and won
And listened in amazement to the hopeful tales they spun.
Their support kept hope alive and I felt understood,
Free to bare my bosom whether feeling bad or good.

The give and take and laughter in my weekly group was grand!
As Father Ben read jokes, cancer cells just wrung their hands.
When, to overcome our stress, our leader led the lion's roar,
Happy T-cells started trampling cancer cells upon the floor.

Some participants faced struggles more insidious than mine.
Brief friendships left fond memories I will cherish for all time.
Their dignity was inspiring, their fortitude redefined
Life, death, and adversity for those they left behind.

For friends who are still fighting, we must not forget to pray.
We must maintain connection and support them in the fray.
To the patrons, keep on giving to this cause so worth the while.
Your gifts have brought much blessing to many in their trial.

When I first came I was frightened; now it's been four years.
With all The Wellness offered, courage triumphed over fear.
Staff and volunteers, I thank you for encouraging me to live.
For the open door to Wellness, heartfelt gratitude I give. 2000

## *NOTHING BUT THE TRUTH*

I Am the Lord, I cannot lie!
My ears are open to your cry;
I died for you, I Am your friend,
I will be with you 'til the end.

Follow Me, even in the dark,
My Spirit will direct your path,
My plans for you are full of hope,
Although you now in darkness grope.

I'll be the husband that you need
And I who sparrows daily feed
Will never leave you begging bread;
You and your children will be fed.

I'll never let you be ashamed,
For you have trusted in My Name;
I Am your Advocate Divine,
I will defend you for you're mine.

When fiery trials around you burn,
I will not from your suffering turn.
I will go with you through the flames,
My love for you will be the same.

So seek and knock and ask of Me
And I will bless abundantly,
Your heart's desire I will give
If for My Glory you will live.

"Delight yourself in the Lord and he will give you the desires of your heart. Commit your ways to the Lord; trust in him and he will do this." Psalm 37:4, 5

## *I BELIEVE*

Your love is everlasting, Lord,
You have declared it in Your Word,
To me You've been a faithful friend,
My wounds You have begun to mend.
When clouds of doubt seem to obscure
Your love for me, so rich, so pure,
Sometimes I fail to realize
I cannot from Your presence hide.

You say You love me as I am,
That only good is in Your plan,
That with me You will always stay,
That You mean every word You say.
Lord, I believe and yet I pray,
Purge me of unbelief today,
Grant me serenity through Your grace,
Put the light of Your peace on my face.

Create within me such a thirst
That I will daily Your Word search,
And in Your presence linger long
Until my heart beats with Your song
Of courage, comfort, love and hope,
Faith and strength to help me cope;
A song of joy that I can share
With hurting people everywhere.

"And without faith it is impossible to please God, because anyone who comes to him must believe that he exists and that he rewards those who earnestly seek him." Hebrews 11:6

# SO WHAT I HAVE NO VALENTINE!

No love romantic is in my life,
For I am nobody's wife.
Nobody's whispering in my ear
Some lie about how much he cares.
No gifts with strings or traps attached,
No dangling carrot I'll *never* catch,
No deadly dance my love to prove,
No headstands one cold heart to move,
No wondering why he's so late,
Nor why my person he berates,
No circular talk to drain my brain,
No more migraines nor chest pains,
No more groveling for what's mine
From some stingy valentine.

Joy and light are in my life,
Don't need to be nobody's wife!
The loving messages I hear
All come from friends who are sincere.
Now I think and dream and feel
And know my feelings are quite real.
My giftedness is in full view.
I do whatever I choose to do.
My hope is high, my heart is free,
God says I'm special and I love me!
So what I have no valentine?
Just look at how much else is mine!

# SISTERS, BEWARE!

Have you ever wondered why
Some men have such a need
To trash our hearts, our homes, our dreams,
And even for their children leave
A legacy of chaos?
This dilemma I have pondered
And have come to understand
That when a man is full of toxic shame,
Cannot forgive or with denial lives,
He can love no one nor can he leave
His self-created cage,
But will inflict his bitterness
On those who come too close.

So sisters, move with caution!
Don't be so quick to give your heart away
Or gauge your worth by any man's attention,
For lips that utter pleasantries today,
Tomorrow may be tirelessly cruel.
In one charmed moment he will steal your heart,
Then crush your spirit with degradations
Designed to bring you down.

You alone are guardian of your heart,
So keep it free from plunder
To live love's joy and wonder;
And if to your own self you would be true,
Seek only for a man worthy of you.

## *I DID DECIDE TO LIVE*

I was already adrift in a sea of pain
When the diagnosis came—
Death of marriage, death of mother,
And then a brand new harbinger of death,
This time my own.
To do or not to do became the question.
Not to do would guarantee a swift demise,
A certain end to suffering.

I had already drunk life's bitter cup,
Felt its poison eat through my existence.
Not to do was easy.
Sometimes tottering on the edge,
I looked both ways, trying to decide.
Then I heard the laughter
Of my son and daughter
And knew I would not leave.

To do would guarantee them
One remaining loyal parent;
And so I did,
I did decide to live.
I asked the Lord for seven years
To see them to adulthood;
Now it has been nearly three.
When seven comes, I'll ask again for me.

## *I HAVE LEARNED*

I have learned as I have lived,
Am still learning, I might add,
That God who made me for His glory
Retains the right to bring into my life
Anything He chooses;
The blessings I so often take for granted
Or fiery trials sent to prove my faith,
For the purifying of my person
Is higher on the list of His priorities
Than my present comfort.
His plan has always been to make me useful,
To extend His love through and beyond myself,
So those still groping in the dark for meaning
May find direction and the hope they seek.

I can choose to waste my suffering
Or profit from its teaching.
I can feed the root of bitterness
Or let forgiveness flow from me.
I can wallow in my woundedness
Or comfort others, as I have been comforted.
I can throw a pity-party in the dark
Or let the light of hope shine forth from me.
I can in anger turn my back on God
Or receive the blessings that dependence on Him brings. 1999

## JOY DEPENDS ON JESUS

We take our cues for happiness
From happenings good or bad.
Gifts received or losses grieved
Make us glad or sad.
While life is unreliable
And people fickle too,
There's one who is unchanging;
He extends true joy to you.

Joy came down at Christmas,
For at the Savior's birth,
Angels proclaimed glad tidings
Of great joy to men on earth.
Jesus lived and died and rose,
Extending grace to all
Who would, in simple faith, believe
And on His mercy call.

He has lived life's disappointments,
Has known betrayal too;
He says, if you abide in Him,
True joy will flow from you—
Joy of sins forgiven,
Joy of hope renewed,
Joy that comes from knowing God
And His love for you.

When we experience conflict
With people and with life,
Joy depends on Jesus,
He is constant in the strife.
So come let us adore Him,
Let's put all else aside,
For when the festive season's done,
His presence will abide. 1999

# HELP OR HINDRANCE

After my trusted helper Clarissa left, Greta offered to help me until I could find someone else. She was being paid, but acted as if she was doing me a favor. She resented being interrupted if I called her to answer a question necessitated by my poor vision. When I asked her to examine some shoes to tell me which ones were worn out or which ones just needed to be cleaned, she shrugged her shoulders and said, "You're the one wearing them!" When I insisted that she clean the ones that needed cleaning, she placed all the dirty shoes on the kitchen counter that she had just washed. I was horrified!

Greta often removed clothes from the dryer while they were still damp, then spread them all over the apartment. I had my own washer and dryer, yet even kitchen towels were spread over the stove burners to finish drying. When I caught her mopping the floor with my Tupperware bowl, I lost it. "What are you doing? This is for my food! Why aren't you using the mop bucket?"

One day I asked Greta to tell me the balance on a credit card statement. She said "zero" and proceeded to rip it up. What madness! After reprimanding her and giving her tape to put it back together. I went to my CCTV. The balance was not zero. I was aghast! Her shenanigans, added to my already overwrought nerves, drove me to drugs, literally. My counselor recommended Paxil for my anxiety.

Brenda arrived decked out as if going on a date. When I asked her to scrub the shower, she complained that her nails and clothes would get "messed up." When she was asked to redo something that was not done well, she threatened to quit. Under emotional stress from other sources, I endured her in silence. My dad had just suffered a massive stroke.

When she threatened to quit for the third time, I kept in mind the date she promised to quit and planned to make it stick. The disappearance of money twice from my wallet solidified that decision. As I signed Brenda's final time sheet, she grumbled about coming out short. Marveling to myself, I said nothing. Would you believe she had the nerve to use me as a reference for her next job?

Casandra became my next paid helper. I call her "Casandra Mañana" and I am "Joy Hoy." In Spanish, "hoy" means "today" and "mañana" means "tomorrow." If something can be put off for the next day, Casandra will do it; not a good match for a type "A" like me. She had a bubbly personality, and I love her dearly, but she drove me "loca." She would do anything as long as my timetable was completely flexible. We were often shopping for groceries at closing time. Because she lived downstairs, her coffee breaks or bathroom breaks could be an hour long. I often went to bed with the smell of bleach as she scrubbed my bathroom at some ungodly hour.

When I reached my wit's end with Casandra and her procrastination, she recommended Marlinda, a very talented woman. There was nothing she couldn't or wouldn't do. She even made some alterations to the dress my daughter wore to her prom. Marlinda spoke very little English, so my Spanish got a working over. A compulsive cleaner, Marlinda loved to throw things out. Every morning she would lunge for the trash, as if it gave her a high. Anything left in the wrong place was game. One day, I purchased a humidifier, hoping it would help my allergies. I wasn't sure if it would work, but knew I could return it. My mistake was to leave the box with all the relevant paperwork in the living room. When I remembered, I was on my way to the gym with Ellen, and Marlinda was at home cleaning.

One day, after repeatedly passing "tornado zone," she must have had an out-of-body moment. Forgetting this was not her house, she scooped up a miscellaneous pile from the floor and took it to the dumpster. Marlinda had regaled me with tales of how she threw her children's clothing, and even the TV, out the window when they annoyed her. That was a family practice for her, but this was my house. We later recovered books, hair ribbons, bed sheets, clothing, etc.

"How could you do that? You are not even responsible for cleaning that room. This is not your house. You cannot throw away things as you please."

A few months later, Agalia complained. Items of clothing were missing from her room, her floor, to be exact. I was slow in believing that Marlinda would have done it again. Of course, she denied it. When I couldn't find a file folder stuffed with important information and kept in a magazine rack under my desk, I was perturbed. It was nowhere in the house. Facing the music, I wrote a letter of dismissal. I was not going on drugs for this one.

I was without a helper and afraid to look for one. The need was still there, but I was not willing to forfeit the feeling of security in my own home. The house was not as clean as before, but I was confident that nothing was being thrown out or stolen, and there were no fire hazards. The real trash sat in the kitchen longer, waiting for my children to rise to the occasion. I ignored what I could and retreated when I couldn't. Eventually Ellen, my trusted friend who had just retired from her nursing career, agreed to be my caregiver. Like any relationship, ours had its moments, but Ellen went above and beyond the call of duty. She stayed with me for 12 years until she retired again.

In some instances, names have been changed to protect the guilty.

# PART 12. PERILS OF PARENTING

## MOM'S CONFESSION

Dear Daughter,

This morning, as I listened to "Focus on the Family", I felt guilty. The topic was "screaming mothers." Dr. James Dobson discussed the damage this does to a child and how intimidating it can be. I am so sorry! I hope you know that, even though I have made this mistake, I do love you very much.

Many things have come into both our lives that make us feel out of control. When the pressure builds, sometimes it seems that my only outlet is to scream. I am not defending screaming, just explaining it. As I listened to Dr. Dobson, the tears were streaming down my face. I was recalling how I felt when my mother yelled at me. Now I was doing the same thing to you.

I love you very much and want to repair the damage. It scares me when you don't do what is right. I want you to become a responsible and mature adult. Forgive me for hurting you in this way. Help me help you by choosing to submit your will to my authority, so that together we can move ahead in a loving relationship. I believe it is the way God wants us to be as mother and daughter. We can both learn from our mistakes!

When I die, I don't want you to remember me as the mother who yelled. I want to be remembered as someone you could talk to about anything; someone who was like velvet over steel, soft and tender, yet strong. That's how I want you to be for your children.

I need you to pray for me every day, so I can become a better mother. Ask God to give me endurance and peace when the going gets rough, and to show you how we can work as a team to make our relationship better. When you recall times I have made you feel sad or unworthy, please forgive me.

Mothers are not perfect. Talk to me about those times. Help me better understand how what I do or say impacts you. I love you so very much.

Mom


## LISTEN TO ME, DAUGHTER

Listen to me, daughter:
You are beautiful and special,
You are gifted and empowered
With inner strength from God.
Your ultimate fulfillment
Comes from spiritual connection
With the one who thus endowed you
With His life and love and grace.

Listen to me, daughter:
Don't ever reach beneath you
To connect with one unworthy,
Just because he is a man!
You're complete in God who made you,
He who never will betray you,
He will give you joy and gladness
As you follow His commands.

Listen to me, daughter:
The real meaning of submission
Is ultimate obedience
To the Lord who knows what's best.
But do not submit to evil
Or abuse from other people,
Set safe limits that will help them
Be the best that they can be.

Listen to me, daughter:
Just delight in whom God made you,
Drink deep of the acceptance
And security He gives.
Use the gifts He's freely given
With a single aim to please Him,
Then from fullness, share with others
Those rich blessings you've received.

## SCHOOL OF HARD KNOCKS

From the school of hard knocks some have chosen to learn
When the wisdom of elders they foolishly spurn.
Yet, none of life's lessons need come this way,
You can hinder much heartache if you heed what God says.

Hear your parents' instruction, obey what you're told,
Treasure correction as silver and gold.
They have lived life before you, know the bumps in the road,
They can warn you of danger, when to stop, where to go.

Some hard knocks are knockouts with ripple effects
That could scar you for life, friends and family affect.
Some trials are errors with a cost far too dear,
For we have just one life with no extras to spare.

There are puddles and potholes, pitfalls to avoid,
The experience of others can serve as a guide.
Observe the results of a deed that's been done,
Appraise what is good, decide what to shun.

In your spirit, determine to choose what is right,
Pursue what is pleasing in God's sight.
Consider your actions before you proceed,
There are good or bad outcomes for every deed.

"Children obey your parents in the Lord; for this is right. 'Honor your father and mother...that it may go well with you and that you may enjoy long life...'" Ephesians 6:1-3

# SNAPSHOTS OF DADDY

Daddy was a hard worker, committed to providing for his household. With just a fourth grade education and a growing family, he struggled for years to find a permanent job. Daddy regularly read the King James Bible and the "Daily Gleaner" (Jamaica's newspaper) in an attempt to improve himself. He worked for some years as a tailor's apprentice. I remember him pressing fabric with the self-heating iron filled with hot coals. He also worked as a waiter at Myrtle Bank Hotel in Kingston, depending heavily on tips to subsidize his salary.

We were delighted to be awakened late at night to share in the delectable leftovers Daddy would bring home. We were not so enthusiastic when he woke us up (before the cock crowed) for family devotions. He expected us to cheerfully sing a hymn, listen to a Scripture reading and pray. Daddy loved to sing! Without television, we spent many evenings singing old gospel hymns. I still sing and play most of those hymns from memory.

In 1967, Daddy immigrated to America in search of greener pastures. A year later, he sent for Mama and the rest of his flock (five of seven children). Grace was attending university. I was working, with no desire to leave Jamaica.

In Boston, Daddy worked two jobs for years. By day, he worked for a camera manufacturer; by night, as an aide in a hospital. He eventually got his GED and bought his first car in his 50's. Uncle Boysie, a Boston realtor, gave Daddy a fixer-upper which became the Walker homestead.

Daddy was a faithful provider of our physical needs, but lacked the ability to connect with his children emotionally. Although generally good-natured, Daddy was a strict disciplinarian, living in an era when parental verbal endearments were rare. Whether I was deliberately disobedient or just made a childish mistake, his scoldings were harsh. I was often declared "good for nothing!"

Constantly judged and criticized, I became an overachiever. I felt unloved and unworthy, desperately needing approval. This drove me, unknowingly, to seek after men who were emotionally unavailable. Unfortunately, I think I married one.

After I started wearing glasses, a single event made me realize that Daddy really did love me. I forgot my glasses one morning and was surprised when Daddy showed up. It was his day off and he took two buses to reach my school. I expected a scolding. Instead, Daddy handed me the glasses with a smile as he said, "You forgot these."

While grieving my divorce, I confronted Daddy on his critical spirit and the legalistic burden he had placed on me as a girl. He had constantly judged my femininity, attributing sinful motives to simple pleasures. His rigidity and negativity had eroded my sense of self, causing me much pain in relationships. Daddy's response surprised me; instead of being defensive, he grieved with me and asked for forgiveness. He had entered marriage and parenting with his own deficiencies (as all of us do); having matured, he humbly acknowledged his failings. I forgave him and, finding healing in the exchange, we developed a deeper bond.

Daddy died the day Agalia graduated from eighth grade. After several strokes near the end of summer 1999, he had been paralyzed and bedridden for ten months. Although unable to fully communicate, Daddy always remembered the words to his favorite hymns when church members visited. After a final stroke, he died peacefully at home.

The children and I spent three weeks in Boston with the family. As we perused his belongings, we were blessed by the many books and tapes indicating Daddy's dogged pursuit of his faith. Daddy served as an elder in his church for 30 years, and was loved by all. He left a rich spiritual legacy, so his memorial service was celebratory. As Daddy often exclaimed, "O Lord, our Lord, how excellent is Thy name in all the earth!"

# FOOTSTEPS OF FAITH

They say that wisdom comes with age,
And even though I am no sage,
I did perceive how much my dad had grown.
His wisdom is seen in the seeds he has sown.
Although I am distressed to see him go,
Today my inner being is aglow
With keen appreciation
For the way he overcame his limitations:
Providing us a home and education;
For faithful commitment to his wife, our mother;
His loving provisions for my sisters and brothers;
The times and ways he bailed us out;
Psalms of praise that flowed from his mouth;
Those moments he opened the Word of God,
Explaining the way of salvation and love;
His fervent prayers on our behalf;
His sense of humor and contagious laugh;
His musical talent, his singing, his smile,
Encouraging conversations across many miles.
The joy he displayed in difficult days
Proved that God's Spirit was with him always.
His suffering had purpose, for even through pain,
He caused each of us to bless God's name.
He has fought the good fight, he has passed the test,
His children have arisen to call him "blessed."
His suffering was a final purification,
In preparation for translocation
Into God's eternal presence,
Where, at this moment, his true essence,
The spirit-man departed from this shell,
Is now completely well,
Enjoying Heaven's bliss,
Free at last from all paralysis.

His patient joy was a testimony to us
Of his unswerving trust in Jesus
To provide complete salvation,
Ultimate hope and consolation.
He has started a new life in a new place,
Truly a work of grace;
A declaration of God's sovereign power
To deliver in the final hour.
In health or sickness, peace or strife,
The torch of faith shone bright in Daddy's life.
His godly example will lead you to grace,
If you follow in the footsteps of his faith.

Dedicated to Claudius James Walker, April 2, 1920-June 8, 2000

## WHERE WOULD I BE?

If the Lord had not rescued me,
Where would I be right now?
If He had dismissed my pleas,
Where would I be right now?
Sorrow would have smothered me,
Torrents swept me away,
Raging waters swallowed me up
If the Lord had not heard me pray.

If help had not come from God,
Where would I be right now?
If I could not trust His care,
Where would I be right now?
His loving kindness is my hope,
His name, my defense and shield,
He gives me rest when I seek His face
When to His control I yield.

Since God is always on my side,
I will sing for joy right now!
He will work all for my good,
As I trust His omnipotent power.
Since I've received such mercy and grace,
To the world I will proclaim
His tender compassion, enduring love,
And with my life, honor His name.

"This is what the Lord says…Fear not…When you pass through the waters, I will be with you; and when you pass through the rivers, they will not sweep over you…For I am the Lord, your God…" Isaiah 43:1-3

## LETTING YOU GO

Eighteen years old, at last you're a man!
All the things you have wished to do now you can.
You just cannot do them here in my house,
Nor can you treat me like peer or spouse.
You may be 18, but we are not equals.
To this adult stuff there's another sequel.
It is not merely age that makes a man,
Wisdom and responsibility are part of the plan.

A real man is responsible from beginning to end.
For his keep, he does not on his mother depend.
So now, I am cutting the apron strings.
You are free to go, you and all your things.
I know I have done the best I could do,
But I guess it's not good enough for you.
Here is your chance to do what you know better,
From now on, it's what you do that will matter.

I've asked God for wisdom again and again,
Have sought good counsel from many wise friends.
God knows the good foundation I have laid.
Have I made mistakes? Oh yes, and I've paid
With pain of disrespect which goes down deep,
And many nights of interrupted sleep;
Hours when I questioned what I had done,
Wondering, "Where on earth did I go wrong?"

Each of us will one day have to pay
For everything we daily do or say,
So dredging up my sins to cover your own
Is not an act the Good Lord will condone.
Since childhood, His Word you have often read.
You may hate my standards, but it is God who said
A mother's wisdom is despised by a fool
And a rebellious heart becomes the devil's tool.

God knows I've always tried to do what's wise,
Perhaps this is a blessing in disguise.
I know I have loved you without condition,
Although, in tough love, I've maintained prohibitions.
You're about to discover true love has its limits.
I will not endorse your destructive habits.
Well, here's to launching you into real life!
Perhaps between us now, there will be less strife.

I am glad you have so many caring friends,
I'm sure what you need they'll give or lend.
Perhaps those for whom you display your charm
Will take you in with outstretched arms.
Perhaps the people you respect so much more
Will help move your baggage away from my door.
You think I am the only problem you have had?
A rare treat is awaiting you, my lad!

The prodigal son thought he had it made.
When all his needy friends around him played
Him for a fool and then walked out,
He was suddenly face to face with a swine's snout.
I cannot sit around to watch you drop,
So in tough love, I'm bringing the bottom up.
Perhaps you will slow down, stop, think, and turn,
Perhaps some wisdom you will sooner learn.


## GRIEF

I work my body until it hurts,
A futile effort to escape the pain,
Obsessing with minutia beyond reason,
Rewinding details of the months just gone:
My son is gone, my heart is torn.
I fast-forward fantasies of the months to come:
He will repent, he will return.
The thought that this may be delusional thinking
Snaps me back to reality and pain,
And so I work and work and work,
Shutting down my brain
To momentarily keep the pain at bay.
My frenzied action is an antidote to grief
Till I must cease.
Then when by night or day
I am again a prisoner
Of my mind's inquisition,
Cries of pain float upward
To mingle with free-falling tears,
Expressions of a heart's unshackled grief.

## CHANGING SEASONS

As Dad lay dying, my son was flying
In the face of maternal authority.
As Dad slowly slipped from manhood
Into his second childhood,
My son was quickly arriving
With no dad to welcome him.
In hormonal confusion
And misguided self-assertion,
He rebelled, despite my frantic pleas.
I had to stand strong, had to play the hand
Life was dealing me.
Dad died, I cried, but grief was put on hold,
As son's rebellion grew more bold.
He went a step too far, now he's gone.
Home is peaceful once again,
Still my heart is filled with pain.
The heat of last season's conflict
Is being cooled by rain, much rain!

"I will turn their mourning into gladness; I will give them comfort and joy instead of sorrow." Jeremiah 31:13

## I AM NOT THE PERFECT PARENT

As a parent, I make choices kids may never understand,
Yet as children they are expected to obey as I command.
I don't have to give a reason for the things I choose to do,
It's my God-ordained assignment, theirs is to obey the rules.

Disobedience may result in pain that hurts both me and them,
For it truly grieves my spirit when instruction they resent.
I can see the road before them, I know where it could lead,
Many problems there await them if my words they do not heed.

243

I make wise and loving choices they can't always understand,
They may argue, scream, protest, and even try to twist my arm.
If I know that their best interest is my top priority,
I will not be swayed by anger or give in to foolish pleas.

When they're being headstrong, I some blessing will withhold.
Till they understand its value, it's a waste to give them gold.
In wisdom, I will test them to discern maturity.
When they are ready to receive it, I will bless them lavishly.

I am not the perfect parent, sometimes I do not have a clue
How to handle the rebellion or the crazy things kids do.
Sometimes my insecurities and weakness wisdom sway,
I give in when I should not, or regret some things I say.

"Parenting is not for cowards," oftentimes the fight is rough.
I must assert authority even when they hate my guts.
But I need to say "I'm sorry" when I know for sure I'm wrong.
I must seek God for wisdom and the faith to keep me strong.

## THE ONLY PERFECT PARENT

God is the only perfect parent, He knows His plan for me,
Though the full scope of His purpose I cannot always see;
If I'm eager to obey Him, to do as He commands,
He will pour out blessings from His gracious, loving hands.

If I am faithful in a little, He will give me so much more!
He desires a yielded vessel into which His love He'll pour.
His plan for me is perfect, not for evil, just for good.
I'd move quickly to obey Him, if His plan I understood.

Like a child I often argue, drag my feet, do my own thing,
Then, when in love He chastens, I resent His discipline.
I forget that He is Sovereign and He answers to no man,
That He'll use drastic measures to fulfill His perfect plan.

If only I would remember how much my God loves me!
If only I would acknowledge His supreme sovereignty!
I would run to do His bidding, I would seek Him every day,
Humbling myself to listen to every word He says.

Lord God, forgive my insolence in questioning Your ways,
For You are the Great Potter while I am just the clay.
Mold me and reshape me according to Your plan,
Forgive me my rebellious ways and guide me with Your hand!


## THE PERFECT HOME

Adam lived in Paradise, the best a home could be.
The Almighty God, his Father, loved him perfectly.
His Father gave him everything his heart could ever need.
For friendship and companionship, He even gave him Eve.
They had a bountiful supply of every kind of food.
They played with all the animals and life was really good!
They both had so much freedom, all of nature was their school.
There was just one restriction, just one simple rule.

God wanted a relationship, not puppets on a string,
Not wind-up toys or robots who couldn't choose a thing.
He wanted them to love Him, as He Himself loved them,
To freely choose obedience in deep respect for Him.
He daily walked and talked with them teaching them His ways.
His voice was music to their ears as they close to Him stayed.
If only they had understood His precept would protect
From danger lurking in a form that they could not suspect.

Before long, there was chaos in this perfect paradise.
Rebellion ruined relations, peace fled from blame and strife.
Adam and Eve were hiding from the one who loved them best;
His Father's heart was broken, when they failed His test.
All of us are children of Adam and of Eve,
For through their disobedience, we were all in sin conceived.
We've each lived in rebellion against the Father's will.
We violate His principles and dishonor His precepts still.

God, the only Perfect Parent, has the only perfect plan.
He conceived the one sure way to rescue sinful man.
To put an end to chaos, to set right what was wrong,
To satisfy His Holiness, He sent His Only Son.
Jesus left us an example of obedience complete
Through His reverent submission, sin and death He did defeat.
His love He is extending to any who will come
Experience true forgiveness, restoring hearts and homes.

Blessing or curse awaits us, depending on our choice.
Our children too must listen and heed the Father's voice.
If as imperfect parents we have pointed them the way,
We must let go and trust God to hold them in His sway.
He has the power to reduce us to the level of a pig,
He will even let us fall into the holes our egos dig.
When from the bottom we look up, His love still reaches down
To pull us from the mire of sin, to save us before we drown.


## *TODAY I CRIED*

Today I cried, releasing grief
To mourn the ending of an era.
Today I cried for unasked questions,
For answers buried with both parents.
Today I cried, with keen awareness of my mortality
Thrust on me by loss and sudden body blow.

Today I cried for love discarded,
Vows violated, a home divided,
The solitary journey of a mom bewildered.
Grief for the son my hands had shown the door.
Today I cried without reserve,
Submerged in the pain of tough love's decision.
Today I cried in unison with truth,
Denial dismissed, yet hope embraced;
Praying for adversity's redemption
In future reconciliation.
Today I cried in volume,
Wringing pain out of my heart.
Today I cried with purpose!

"This is what the Lord says: Restrain your voice from weeping and your eyes from tears, for your work will be rewarded." Jeremiah 31:16

## TOMORROW

May tomorrow, Lord, be better
Just because I cried today.
May I rise up from my weeping
To understand Your ways.
May I die to my ambitions
And the need to have control.
Then in place of my desires, put Your own.

Bend your ear to my petition,
Lord, supply the grace I need.
For Your wisdom and perspective,
Lord, to You I intercede.
May Your resurrection power
Follow the cross I bear this hour.
Bring Your healing once again into our lives.

In my grief, make my heart hopeful
As to You I entrust my son,
Knowing, Lord, that You are faithful
To complete what You've begun.
May the seeds I've sown in sorrow
Yield the fruit of joy tomorrow.
Let me then enjoy the labor of my hands.

Put my tears into your bottle
When my soul cries out to You.
My anxieties please settle,
Send Your peace to see me through.
You are Mercy and Compassion,
Lord, You know my heart's condition.
Draw my child back from his wandering to Your arms.

Mold the circumstance of his life;
Make it all work out for good.
Turn his heart around to trust in You
Completely, as he should.
Heal the soul wounds he is bearing;
Show him You are always caring.
Bring back joy into his heart and to our lives. 2000

"Those who sow with tears will reap with songs of joy." Psalm 126:5

## *HELP ME SMILE AGAIN*

Lord, I do not understand
Why my foolish heart tries to run,
Thinking that I can escape
Your deep love for me.

Lord, there's so much pain inside,
I feel that I just want to run and hide,
Yet, there is no place where I can go
That Your love won't follow me.

When fear and failure come my way,
When disappointments mar my day,
When I am feeling all alone,
When life's vicissitudes overwhelm,
Lord, give to me sustaining grace,
Look with favor on my tear-stained face,
Come hold me here in all my pain,
Help me smile again.

Help me comprehend
You are the only one who can
Forgive me all the wrong I've done
And love me anyway.
Lord, help me now to realize
That You are always by my side,
That You will heal my heart once more,
Help me smile again.

"Where can I go from your Spirit? Where can I flee from your presence? If I go up to the heavens, you are there; if I make my bed in the depths, you are there. If I rise on the wings of the dawn, if I settle on the far side of the sea, even there your hand will guide me, your right hand will hold me fast." Psalm 139:7-10

## PURPOSE IN MY PAIN

One day, much bewildered about the way life had turned out,
I questioned God's doings, what all this heartache was about.
I had missed the bigger picture for right then I could not see
Everything that happened was not just about me.
I'd heard God uses pain to speak to more than just one man,
So I asked Him then to help me better understand His plan.

His answer soothed my heartache, for I understood that day
There is purpose in my suffering. This is what I heard Him say:
"Adversity reminds you that you are weak and small,
That you cannot live without Me, but on My strength must fall.
When I give you power to stand the test life's trials bring,
When from your broken heart a song of joy you dare to sing,
Those who are listening will know that your God truly lives.
Then you can speak to others of the comfort that I give."

"I love the Lord, for he heard my voice; he heard my cry for mercy. Because he turned his ear to me, I will call on him as long as I live." Psalm 116:1, 2


## SWEET REVENGE

You think me dull, antiquated and square,
That I haven't a clue what's happening out there.
That I ask any questions really frustrates you.
That I dare to say no exasperates too!

You think I am a blubbering fool
For insisting you go to church and school.
You're so lucky I let you go out at all,
For I'm only a killjoy after all!

You wish I would chill and just let you be
Like your other friends, you just want to be free
To come and go and do as you please.
From parental bondage you want your release.

You scream in my face that you think I am nuts,
You'll kill yourself and you hate my guts,
Then, a few moments later, with outstretched hand,
And no sign of contrition, my money demand.

You teenagers are certainly tripping
On raging hormones and screws that are missing.
Do you know there are kids who wish someone would care
Enough to say, "That is dangerous, dear?"

I care for your safety and love you too much,
That's why I make all this terrible fuss.
I will cramp your style if it keeps you alive,
I do want to see you grow and thrive.

If you don't get too crazy, someday you'll be old
Like me, then my wisdom to you will be gold.
I will be right here when you come to inquire
About what to do with the children you've sired.

Revenge will be sweet, I'll be having much fun
As you go bananas restraining your son
From behavior you know full well could destroy
Or impede the progress of that young boy.

When your kids call you foolish and old-fashioned too,
I'll stifle a chuckle and wink at you.
You will have grown sane, and I, so much wiser!
No more will you deem me a stupid old geezer.


## USE MY PAIN

May life's painful lessons be of some use, somehow,
To others I encounter to help them as they grow.
May my failures be productive in the lives of some I meet,
Protecting them from pitfalls which have ensnared my feet.
May I reflect the wisdom from all my blunders gained,
And may discretion guide them from such blunders to refrain.
For wisdom can be gathered by heeding wayward steps,
And choosing not to follow can save from sad regrets.

For some who, by example, have taught us what to shun,
By their own foolish choices, alas, have been undone!

"For the waywardness of the simple will kill them, and the complacency of fools will destroy them; but whoever listens to me (wisdom) will live in safety and be at ease...For the Lord gives wisdom, and from his mouth comes knowledge and understanding. He holds victory in store for the upright...then you will understand what is right and just and fair—every good path. For wisdom will enter your heart and knowledge will be pleasant to your soul." Proverbs 1:32, 33; 2:7-10

# PART 13. REIGN OF TERROR

## NEW DOWNPOUR

Hoping that 2001 would be a new beginning, a year in which I would recover joy, I began to lift my head above the flood waters of 2000. The poem "Sweet Revenge" was me trying to find humor in the pain. My son was living with his father. Child support had to be adjusted, so I was dialoguing with my lawyer again. While dreading the legal ordeal and still smarting over the alienation between my son and me, I received a phone call from Paul.

"Grace is dead!"

"What?" I screamed. "Are you serious?"

Grace had been recovering from surgery where a portion of her colon had been removed. Later, we learned that she had been battling colon cancer for five years. This means we both had been fighting different cancers at the same time. She had kept information from us, so her death was a shock.

Grace visited Daddy a few months before he died. Faith remembers her final farewell to Daddy as very emotional. She had promised to see him in Heaven, if not again on Earth. While she was in Boston (in April 2000), I called Grace from California, unaware it would be our last conversation. It was almost a year later when Paul called with the news that Grace had suffered a heart attack.

Before leaving for Jamaica, I visited my oncologist.

"How are you?"

"You don't want to know," I replied with a heavy sigh. I told him about the conflict with my son, my father's death, the impending legal hassles, and the recent news of my sister's death.

"There is too much on your plate!" (I had heard those words before.) "You need some help. Let me see if the psychiatrist is available. She may be able to give you something before you leave for Jamaica."

The psychiatrist, after listening to me emote, commended my courage and recommended a drug called Effexor.

"I have tried several antidepressants before," I protested. "I do not want to sleep my life away or live like a zombie." I listed the meds I had tried. The most recent, after just one month, left me unable to lift my head from the pillow.

A visiting nurse had been coming to my house periodically to clean my Groshong catheter. She came unexpectedly one Sunday morning. It was Mother's Day. I had planned to go to church but couldn't get out of bed. Concerned about my extreme lethargy, she promised to check on me later. Alarmed, I quit cold turkey that day with no intentions of ever using another mood-altering medication. The psychiatrist assured me that Effexor was different; it wasn't addictive and was in an extended-release capsule. I decided to try it.

When Grace and I were young, many people thought we were twins. She was the only member of our family who had not migrated to the United States, though she visited occasionally. The last time I had been to Jamaica was in 1977, for Grace's wedding. Now I was returning 23 years later for her burial. Grace was four months shy of her 52nd birthday, and I was 53. Starting the antidepressant before going to the funeral was a timely move. Despite the deep sorrow in losing my sister, I embraced the joy of reuniting with family and friends I hadn't seen in years. All my recent traveling had been about death and dying. Who would be next?

On returning home, I found a letter from my lawyer. It was Saturday and I was scheduled to be in court the following Monday. I panicked. My ex and his new wife were eager to adjust the child support, but ignored the fact that he owed me money. I was grieving, and going to court again was traumatic. Although I had regularly labeled in Braille all receipts and correspondence, it was a nightmare putting it together, finding and then losing information repeatedly. I was a nervous wreck until my friend Nichole rescued me.

My attorney was not able to be in court that day and his proxy did not know the whole history of the case. The judge ran through proceedings rather quickly, ignoring the money owed to me.

Adjustments were made, and an additional $50 would be deducted from the check each month for the balance due my ex. It was lunch time. The judge hurried out the door without saying when the deduction would stop. I was disheartened. Even the court clerk agreed that I got a bad deal. The overpayment and unpaid medical bills were never recovered.

"Why, God?" I pondered. "This wasn't fair." Frequently, especially when Agalia was in college, I was tempted to go after him for that money. Each time the temptation came, I decided the following.

What happened in court did not surprise God. Was it unfair? Yes. Life is unfair. I could go back to court, but God allowed this outcome for a purpose. Starting another legal battle was not worth the emotional or financial cost. I would probably pay the lawyer more than I would gain for my effort. As a cancer survivor, I needed to minimize stress and avoid toxic situations and people as much as possible. This outcome is a constant reminder of God's promise to take care of His children. I stand amazed at His faithfulness.

A few months later, like every other American, I was stunned by the mind-boggling terror attacks on the World Trade Center. The news seemed surreal until the personal stories started emerging. Fortunately, under the influence of Effexor, I did not absorb the full emotional impact. Thank God for that! From my sofa, I spent many mesmerizing hours watching TV in shocked incredulity. Over the next few months, I wrote three poems in an attempt to process the inexplicable horror.

Overweight and stressed, I was challenged by my sister's death to get moving. Life is unpredictable and death is certain, but I wasn't ready to go. When I discovered that my HMO provided a free gym membership, I jumped at the opportunity. Joining a gym, I started attending "Silver Sneakers," a fitness program for seniors and people with disabilities. I weighed 218 lbs. and losing that weight became a priority. Determined to extricate Joy from this quagmire of death and dying, I started moving. Fifteen years later, despite the ups and downs of weight loss, I have lost and kept off 70 lbs.

## *HOW WILL I BE REMEMBERED?*

I cannot choose when I will go, nor in what circumstance,
But I can choose how I will live and other lives enhance.
I realize my sojourn here is temporary too,
So I must ponder carefully the things I say and do.

How will I be remembered by those I leave behind?
As loved ones filter memories, what treasures will they find?
What precious recollections will they cherish long?
Kind words aptly spoken, a deed well done, a cheerful song?

Will benevolence be remembered by those who were in need?
Will hope have been revived by my sowing friendship's seed?
Will a searching heart find answers in wisdom freely shared?
Will faltering faith grow stronger because I really cared?

Will truth spoken in genuine love restore a wayward soul?
Will my liberal forgiveness make a broken spirit whole?
If I sinned against another, was I quick to admit my wrong?
Did I dare stand for justice, though I stood against the throng?

Did lessons gleaned from failure make me better grow?
Then, for another's weakness, did I compassion show?
When I walked through fiery trials that seemed to have no end,
Did my friends know it was Jesus who supplied my strength?

Was someone's life made fruitful when I took time to pray?
Did someone find the Savior because I showed the way?
Will I in some small way have made this world a better place
By being a channel of God's love, His beauty and His grace?

Dedicated to Grace Marie Walker Gordon (July 19, 1949-March 14, 2001)

## *ME AGAIN LORD*

Me again Lord, down on my knees!
It's for Your comfort that I plead.
I seem to stand on shifting sand.
All I can do is grasp Your hand.
There is so much I can't control,
So many storms sweep o'er my soul.
Lord, I will never make it through
If I don't put my trust in You.

Help me to understand Your way,
Teach me to trust You day by day,
Give me a song in darkest night,
Send me your peace, steer me aright.
Please hold my hand, don't let me go.
You are the only Friend I know
Who will be there through fire and flood.
You are my Savior and my God!

For Your great glory I was made,
Remind me, O Lord, when I'm afraid,
That having suffered much for me,
You offer me true empathy.
When Your whole purpose I can't see,
I know You know my destiny.
For all these tears I'll gain a crown,
With joy, at Your feet, I'll lay it down.

"Let us then approach the throne of grace with confidence, so that we may receive mercy and find grace to help us in our times of need." Hebrews 4:16

## *THIS PRESENT ALARM*

A fire alarm is a warning bell
That lets us know all is not well.
It is time to send a SOS,
It isn't time for paralysis.
So you pick up the phone, call 9-1-1,
Then out of danger to safety run.

On 9/11, 2001,
From apathy our nation sprang.
As airplanes plummeted from the sky,
And Twin Towers tumbled before our eyes,
Violent men snatched loved ones away
With no regard for the plight of their prey.

Though our country mourns for thousands gone,
We can't let the terrorists think they won.
America's enemies plot her demise
For the Lady Liberty they despise.
Justice is needed, yet war brings more dread.
Other loved ones could soon be dead.

This present alarm should urge us to call
On the Sovereign God who rules over all.
While the fear of man is a trap and a snare,
God's perfect love casts out all fear.
A spirit of dread He did not give to us,
But a spirit of power and love and trust.

Blessed is the nation that hopes in the Lord,
That seeks His protection, takes Him at His Word.
He promised to make all things work for good
To those who reverence Him as God.
If we seek for mercy and help from His hand,
He will do as He promised and heal our land.

"If my people, who are called by my name, will humble themselves and pray and seek my face and turn from their wicked ways, then I will hear from heaven, and I will forgive their sin and will heal their land." 2 Chronicles 7:14

## AMERICA UNDER ATTACK

Jumbo jets transformed into weapons of mass destruction
Deployed by convoluted minds to terrorize America at home,
Slam into New York's Twin Towers.
Lives vaporize before our eyes, as exploding jet fuel
Lights human torches.
As flaming fusillade and burning bodies fall
Upon the unsuspecting,
Panicking people press into crowded stairwells
Trying to get out.
In frenzied fear, some jump out.
On cell phones, others verbalize their love
For the last time.
In face of common danger, strangers become friends,
Risking their lives for neighbors.
Brave police and firemen courageously rush in,
Selfless in their commitment, heroes on the move
Dying as they had lived.
The nation gasps in unison as the Twin Towers tumble,
New York's giants defeated in their prime.
Spontaneous cries of "O my God!" slide from stunned mouths.
Plumes of black smoke merge with the desultory dust of death
Shrouding the landscape in terror.
Shards of splintered glass, twisted molten steel,
Tons of smashed concrete, live electrical wires
And furnishings turned firewood
Form a blazing funeral pyre for thousands of mangled bodies,
And innocence gone forever.

## *AMERICA MOURNS*

America mourns her children lost,
Moving between fury, fear and sorrow,
Praying without political correctness:
"God Bless America!"
Her heart is broken but still beats
With passion, fortitude and faith,
Stirred by the heroes who fought back
Undaunted in the face of death.

Stories of strong survivors
And tales of tireless rescuers
Remind her that from evil God brings good.
Her sons and daughters now unite
To honor the liberty we love,
Aware that life at best is brief,
That how we live and memories we leave
Are really all that matter,
That God alone can bless America now!

"…You are my refuge in the day of disaster." Jeremiah 17:17

## **SILVER LINING**

It was October 2001, time for Silver Saturday, a celebratory workshop at The Wellness Community for breast cancer survivors. I was almost there. December 19th would be my five-year anniversary. Hallelujah! It was awesome as I stood with fellow survivors while others applauded. It had been a tumultuous five years, but I survived cancer and everything else!

In December 2001, I was declared "in remission," the words every cancer survivor lives for. Now I would need to see my oncologist just once each year and, of course, continue to get a yearly mammogram. I breathed a sigh of relief and a prayer. May the news be this good every year!

"Praise the Lord, O my soul; all my inmost being, praise his holy name. Praise the Lord, O my soul, and forget not all his benefits—who forgives all your sins and heals all your diseases, who redeems your life from the pit and crowns you with love and compassion, who satisfies your desires with good things so that your youth is renewed like the eagle's." Psalm 103:1-5

# PART 14. RECLAIMING JOY

## COME CELEBRATE WITH ME

Friend, come celebrate with me another year.
Have no care about a gift, just you be here!
Special times I spend with you are far more dear.
Things tangible will soon wear out or need repair,
But memories we make with friends last many years.
Come, be merry, eat a lot and laugh aloud!
Just for this day, we'll banish care or threatening cloud.
Whatever tomorrow may bring, right now let's sing
And make new joyful memories, my friend! (Birthday 54)

## BIG SURPRISE

I had just returned from a visit to the neurosurgeon regarding a bulging disc and pinched sciatic nerve. I shared the surgeon's reluctance to do back surgery. The benefit might not outweigh the risks. Leery about too much medication, I was left with little choice except to grin and bear it. Exiting the car slowly, I said to Ellen, "I suppose I'll have to resort to the meds when I can't grin." The cumulative effect of several falls over the years had contributed to severe chronic back pain. Climbing the stairs daily to my second floor apartment exacerbated the discomfort.

Just then, my daughter darted through the security gate shouting excitedly, "Mom, Mom, there's a big surprise waiting for you inside. You won't believe it!"

"What is it?" I asked.

"I'm not going to tell you. You will have to see for yourself. Hurry!" I mounted the stairs as fast as my aching legs would allow. As I entered the front door, a husky voice greeted me.

"Hey Sis! What a gwaan?" I shrieked with delight as my brother Danny and I embraced, rocking back and forth. Danny's girlfriend,

Darlene, Agalia and Avizi (yes, Avizi had come back to live with me and we were on much better terms) were all laughing too.

"This is really a BIG surprise! You were right, Agalia," I giggled. Danny was 6'3" and weighed at least 275 lbs.

"What breeze blow you in, man? It's so good to see you!"

When any of my siblings and I get together, much clowning goes on. We laugh until we're in stitches. This time was no different. It was refreshing because, as a single mom dealing with limited finances and argumentative teenagers, life wasn't so funny sometimes. Besides, we had no family in California to provide occasional relief. When he told me his son, also Danny, had a baby, I remarked with amusement, "Oh, so now I have to call you Granny Danny!" There was another outburst of hilarity.

Danny and Darlene were vacationing in San Diego and drove up to Los Angeles to surprise us. My children were thrilled when he handed each of them some cash. After much chatter and joviality, we all decided to go shopping. Agalia needed a dress for the prom and her favorite uncle was treating. Danny, Darlene, Agalia and I piled into the rental car and headed for the Mall. I assumed we were only going for Agalia's dress; that would have been pleasing enough for me.

When Agalia went off with Darlene to find her dress, Danny decided we would do some shopping for me. The care with which Danny helped me shop was heartwarming. He was scooping up items without regard for price, dismissing my nervous inquiries. As I tried on clothes, Danny kept handing me more items over the door. When we checked out, I was stunned! Maybe $300 is no big deal to some, but it was to this single mom.

"You made me feel special," I murmured, touched by his kindness.

"Well, you are special!" Danny responded, putting his arms around me. "It isn't that I have so much, but I know you need it. Happy Mother's Day!" It was the Tuesday before Mother's Day, but that had not been on my mind.

When we caught up with the girls, they showed us the dress Agalia had selected. I groaned and looked at Danny.

"Can you handle it?"

"Yes, it's okay," Danny nodded. The dress was a rosy pink satin overlaid with a sheer black chiffon that opened in front. The bodice was strapless with sparkling rhinestones across the neckline. It was not available in her size, so the saleswoman arranged to order it from another store.

After shopping, we went to a Chinese restaurant. "Too bad Avizi left with his friend," I remarked. "We will have to take him a doggie bag." We chuckled as Danny teased his niece about being vegetarian. She nibbled tofu and vegetables while the rest of us devoured beef, chicken, pork and shrimp. It didn't bother us a bit that she scorned our carnivorous inclinations.

Before Darlene and Danny left, he handed me the money for Agalia's dress. When Darlene also offered me cash to do her hair for the prom, I was overwhelmed with gratitude.

"Whatever breeze blew you in," I chuckled, "I hope it keeps blowing this way." As grateful as I was to them, my gratitude overflowed even more toward God. He always supplies my needs. Everything belongs to Him, so He can use anyone willing to reflect His heart of love and generosity.

"Mom, isn't God good? I have been praying for a miracle because I knew you didn't have the money for the prom. Now He has given far more than I could ask or think, just like it says in the Bible (Ephesians 3:20). It is even more amazing that God cares about a little thing like the prom." My daughter was mature enough to see the prom as "little" in the scheme of things. I was impressed.

"Great is the Lord and most worthy of praise...One generation will commend your works to another...They will celebrate your abundant goodness." Psalm 145:3, 4, 7

*Joy Walker*

## HE WILL NOT FAIL ME

God never needs to change His mind,
He is not limited by time.
There's nothing that He cannot do
So all his promises are true.

Refrain:
He does no wrong, He cannot lie,
His holy nature He will not deny.
My faith in Him is quite secure.
He will not fail me, I am sure!

His wrath for sin is just as true
As His deep love for me and you.
On one condition He relents,
If in contrition we repent.

In Him I find my strength and joy
When cares of earth my soul annoy.
He understands my every need,
So when perplexed, to Him I'll plead.

All He has done was for my good,
Even when I have not understood.
His plans for me are good and pure.
He will not fail me, I am sure!

"The Lord is faithful to all his promises and loving toward all he
has made." Psalm 145:13b

## MOSES

Moses grew up as a choice Prince of Egypt,
Yet sensed something missing even as a small child.
He took no delight in the pleasures of Egypt,
His heart yearned for something far more worthwhile.

His mom had regaled him when he was much younger
With tales of her God and His covenant plan.
Moses remembered and pondered her stories
And wondered if he would be God's special man.

When Moses was forty, he witnessed the suffering
Imposed on his kinsmen by Pharaoh's demand.
He saw an Egyptian opposing a Hebrew,
He slew and concealed him 'neath Egypt's hot sand.

He thought it his duty, leaned on his own wisdom,
Forgetting that vengeance belongs to the Lord.
Evil for evil creates a conundrum
Which can be avoided by heeding God's Word.

He thought no one knew, but the news soon reached Pharaoh,
Who sought to kill Moses for slaying that man.
Moses had failed and his heart filled with terror.
Dismayed, disillusioned, from Egypt he ran.

God's plan was not sidetracked by Moses' big failure,
He still meant to use him, but in His own time.
From riches to rags, without country or kinsmen,
He knew not that, through him, God's glory would shine.

For forty years, he tended sheep in the desert
While growing in patience and humility.
Then God called to him from the midst of the fire,
In majestic display of divine purity.

267

When God challenged Moses to rescue His people
From Pharaoh's oppressive and treacherous hand,
Afraid to face Pharaoh, he argued, "I *sttu-stutter*,
*Ppplease* send someone else. I am not the right man."

He lost the debate. God's purpose is sovereign.
Moses told Pharaoh, "Let my people go!"
High-minded Pharaoh thought Moses was trifling.
To show who was boss, God put on a great show.

When it was done, Israel had left Egypt
And Pharaoh's whole army lay dead in the sea.
Moses knew then that a heart fully yielded
Could show to the world God's divine sovereignty.

If you are longing for purpose and meaning,
Ask God for His wisdom, the plan He designed.
Then when you catch glimpses of His nobler purpose,
Don't try to out-step God, but wait for His time.

If now in the desert, learn patience from suffering,
Let hardship and failure your nature refine.
Acknowledge your weakness, then go forth in God's strength.
Then through you, to others, His glory will shine.

Dedicated to Agalia on her graduation from high school


## EMPTY NEST PRAYER

A brand new phase of life has just begun for me today.
The nest is empty, for the fledglings both have flown away.
My feelings are conflicted, though for the most part I am glad.
You've been with me through much, I've no reason to be sad.

There are so many things I have not had much time to do.
Even times with You, Lord, sometimes have been so few.
There are no more excuses, all the turmoil has subsided.
Now there's time to seek You with attention undivided.

Spouse and children are all gone, but You will never go.
Although at times I'll feel alone, I know it isn't so.
Lord, You know all that I need, I'll trust You to provide.
In my fearful moments You'll be right here by my side.

Guide me through this season, show me what's in store.
Where my steps will take me from today, I am not sure.
I know I'm far from useless, that there's more for me to do.
Of all the gifts You've given, show me which ones to pursue.

Grant me Your perspective even as I'm growing old;
As I fight the good fight, give me courage to be bold.
Bring me those who need Your love to fill their emptiness.
Give me a new design as I rebuild my empty nest.


## I'M GOING TO JAMAICA

I'm going to Jamaica this year. Can I afford it? Who cares! I'm tired of having my flying dictated by death and dying—Mama, Daddy, Grace. It's time to change the pace. So now I'm flying for Joy! Oh boy! I definitely will be going in April. Why then? I will be 57. It's high time to celebrate without measure the long-awaited pleasure of walking the shores of my native land, hand in hand with old friends, recalling our youthful days and all the ways life has blessed us. My excitement is growing, because I'm definitely going to Jamaica this year! 2005

# JOY IN JAMAICA

In December 2004, with both children out of the house, I accepted an invitation to a reunion with cousins to be convened in Florida. I relished the idea of taking a trip for pure fun. The event was hosted by Ruth and Roy, who were celebrating their 30th wedding anniversary and Ruth's 50th birthday. On December 26th, we watched in disbelief news of the Sumatra earthquake and ensuing tsunami. I learned later that, hours before the cataclysmic events, elephants and birds were seen fleeing to higher ground, while unsuspecting people gathered seashells on the seashore. Thousands of people perished but few animal carcasses were found.

Ruth's sisters, Claudette and Marcia, closest to my age, were the oldest of Aunt Darling's eight children. As a city girl, I always enjoyed visiting them in the country and catching crayfish from Wag Water River near their house. The girls asked me when I would visit Jamaica again. With my yearning for home awakened, I decided to celebrate my next birthday on the island.

At the Gospel Hall where I received my early Christian training, I had attended Sunday school, sang soprano in the choir and in a girls' trio, and played piano for church services. On this visit, I was pleased to learn that two youngsters whom I had taught to play piano by ear, were now involved in music ministry. At the request of a church elder, I counseled a mother and daughter who were hurting from a recent divorce. I believe they received some measure of comfort.

To my surprise, I was invited, along with a former classmate, to be a guest on a Christian talk show broadcast on a local television station. We discussed the role of godly faith in coping with life's challenges. Addressing the assembly of girls at my former high school was also an unanticipated privilege and pleasure, although it evoked a not so happy memory. In my senior year, I was a prefect (student monitor) with varying duties, including reading Scripture to the entire school when we gathered for morning worship.

One day, I opened the Bible before 750 girls and teachers. To my dismay, I couldn't see the words! Petrified, I quickly deliberated my way out of the dilemma; from memory, I recited Psalm 23, then fled the platform. The headmistress knew that wasn't the chosen text, but said nothing. I felt like a fool, but stuffed my feelings. Almost 40 years later, I was addressing a similar assembly, this time speaking with confidence about my vision loss.

Challenging these young girls with the poem "Listen to Me, Daughter," I warned them against the folly of thinking some boy or man would make them happy. I encouraged them to take their education seriously, pursue God's plan for their lives, and strive toward their full potential. It was gratifying to think I could make a positive impact on so many lives.

Though a native islander, I had a fear of water and had never gone rafting. Enrolling in water aerobics class had removed some of that fear. Still unable to swim, I was a little scared; nevertheless, I decided to go rafting on the Rio Grande in Ocho Rios. Drifting along to the sound of Calypso music floating on the air was exhilarating. When we reached shallow waters, Marcia and I slid in and splashed around. I was so proud of myself! I went rafting and have pictures to prove it.

It was nostalgic to spend time with extended family of varying ages. I visited former classmates and teachers, including Mrs. Urquhart, who had encouraged me to learn Braille. We drove past familiar neighborhoods, but couldn't linger long in some places that had become unsafe. My cousins advised me to avoid the area where I had discovered those Braille bumps. Good thing I listened. The TV evening news reported a standoff between police and gangsters that had transpired that very day.

My cousins, Marcia, Claudette and Mardell, rounded up some "old" friends and threw me a surprise birthday party. I savored some native cuisines: ackee and salt fish, mackerel and run-down, bammy, breadfruit, rice and peas, jerk chicken, jerk pork, ginger beer and patties.

Claudette informed me that she would be getting married in December. She had kept the secret from me in Florida, afraid I'd change my mind about coming in April. It was exciting news and I was having such a good time, I decided to return.

Agalia accompanied me in December. It was her first time visiting my island home and meeting the extended family. My mother's only remaining brother, Uncle Eddie, was delighted to meet her. My cousin John drove us through Content and Cavaliers where my parents grew up. My paternal grandparents, Joseph and Albertha Walker, are buried on the property in Content.

We also visited Emancipation Park (the most popular public park in Kingston), dedicated to the memory of Jamaica's liberation from slavery in 1838. After purchasing trinkets from Victoria Craft Market, we enjoyed a fish fry at the beach. On Christmas morning, we attended an early church service followed by the cousins' traditional Christmas breakfast at the Hilton Hotel. Of course, it wouldn't be Christmas in Jamaica without sorrel, our traditional Christmas drink, and our famous rum-soaked fruitcake.

Claudette and Maurice had an interactive wedding. Except for the singing of a hymn or two, rising for the bride's entrance and the couple's exit at the end, wedding guests usually sat quietly. This wedding was different.

Four lovely ladies, dressed in beautiful turquoise dresses, took delicate dancing steps towards the front of the church. They perched themselves on stools festooned with ribbons and bows of yellow and turquoise. Claudette's young nieces, adorned in yellow, scattered flower petals down the aisle. Her nephews unrolled the white carpet in preparation for the bride's entrance.

As Marcia, Claudette's sister and matron of honor (wearing yellow), made her grand entrance, a "Wow!" went up from the crowd. I thought the bride had entered. The congregation was pressing into the aisles in eager anticipation. The excitement was electrifying as Maurice walked toward his bride. She approached him singing. He responded in kind. With gusto, the audience joined in the last line of each verse. The most unusual part of the ceremony was when the minister asked, "Who gives this woman to be married?" A spontaneous and jubilant outburst of "We do!" went up from the audience.

Claudette and Maurice were a mature couple whose parents had passed on. It was Claudette's first wedding. Seven candles were lit, in memory of deceased parents and siblings from both families, followed by a moment of silence in their honor.

Claudette, Sunday school superintendent for many years, had invested in the lives of countless children; she was dearly loved by the congregation. It was evident in their enthusiasm. While the bride and groom signed the register, the dancing bridesmaids made their graceful moves, thrilling the audience. No one missed any of the action, except me, but someone kept me up to speed with a minute-by-minute commentary.

This wedding was worth the cost of my airplane ticket. It was such a joyous occasion! Claudette later sent me a close-up photo of yours truly, arms stretched out and eyes bulging, attempting (with all the other single ladies) to catch the bouquet. Can't say I didn't try!

A few years later, I tried again. Kitty and Brent were both blind and I was one of many blind/visually impaired guests attending their wedding. Imagine my surprise and pleasure when the bouquet landed in my outstretched arms. Lest you think I have aspirations toward a wedding of my own, let me set the record straight. It's not so easy to catch a good man, so that's not on my bucket list.

## YOU DID IT AGAIN

O my Lord, You did it again!
Showed me my suffering was not in vain.
All these years and full circle I've come
Back to where the brokenness began;
Back where You first claimed me,
Placed Your stamp of love upon me;
But in my brokenness I wandered,
Slipping my hand from Yours.

Biting the bait of counterfeit love,
I added brokenness to brokenness.
While I floundered in the dark,
You never gave up on me
But held out Your hand of mercy
Till I could grasp it again.
Now at rest in Your embrace,
I ponder Your unfathomable love
And how You use my woundedness to heal
Others now broken as I was.


## JOY IN SUFFERING

After wrestling with the idea for some time, I was ready for breast reconstruction nine years after the mastectomy. My friend, Julie, had double breast reconstruction in 2004. Motivated by her success, I arranged surgery for July 18th, 2005.

Ellen and Agalia accompanied me to Huntington Hospital. Shortly after arriving, I was met by Maurine and Sonya, who planned to keep vigil for the duration. Maurine and her sister Margaret had also kept vigil during my mastectomy in 1997. I said my goodbyes, oblivious to what was ahead. I remember being rolled on the gurney toward the operating room on Monday morning. I awoke on Friday evening surrounded by several friends and family. Faith had flown in from Boston, a huge surprise.

A tube in my throat inhibited my speech. I was gesticulating wildly in an attempt to communicate. Alas, Joy could not be heard! My friend, Jasmine, practical as always, gave me a pad and pen, but my handwriting was illegible. My frustration grew. Still unaware of all that had transpired, I was stunned as the revelation came in bits and pieces.

Complications had necessitated a blood transfusion. Blood clots had developed, threatening the success of the operation. To top it all, a full-blown asthma attack had landed me on a ventilator. I had been in the ICU for four days. The hospital was inundated with phone calls on my behalf. When I was able to speak again, no one could shut me up. They kept telling me to save my strength, but, every Walker is a talker, so I was making up for lost time.

When I was out of danger, just about everyone started out, "You scared us" or "Don't you scare us like that again." My response was, "Only two people were not scared. God wasn't, because nothing takes Him by surprise; and me, I didn't have a clue." My friend Earl teased, "What's new about that?" Low blow!

Unable to climb the stairs to my second floor apartment, I spent two weeks in a convalescent hospital. My roommate, 79, had undergone open-heart surgery. Surprisingly, she had spent one day in the ICU, while I had spent four. My recovery was rapid. Ruth said I motivated her to get out of bed. Even the staff was amazed by my daily improvement.

One day the physical therapist failed to show up. Sitting in my wheelchair next to Ruth, I started moving my legs and arms. Giggling, she began mimicking my every move. We were having our own PT class. I thought of Mama, who died at 79.

The Sunday before leaving, I sat down at the Steinway piano in the lobby. I was told that no one had played it in a long time. A few people sitting close by immediately showed their appreciation. Soon I felt like the Pied Piper of Hamlin, as wheelchairs scurried from their rooms drawn by the music. My audience grew, as did their delightful cries.

"Goody, goody, goody!" cried a man as he clapped his hands.

"That one brought tears to my eyes," a woman sniffled. "I never thought I would hear such beautiful music here on a Sunday morning."

"I didn't know you could play," the activity director cooed with delight. "You will have to come back and play for us." A nurse who hailed from Hungary came to my room later. "You are a beauty pianist," she remarked in her broken English. "Everybody loved it. You are a great success when everybody loves it."

I felt real joy. One of God's gifts to me had again brought cheer to many. Is that not the essence of fulfillment? God is still on His throne. Whatever tomorrow may hold, I have the assurance that He will make it work for good.

Just weeks after my surgery, I was stunned by the news of Hurricane Katrina and the devastation left in her wake. As with 9/11, the personal stories moved my heart. A man wept for his wife, swept from his arms by the raging water. A woman agonized over her missing mother-in-law, who had been in a hospital. A cop committed suicide after his wife and daughter drowned in their home; he had ignored their pleas to evacuate. Little ones were separated from parents, some too young to identify themselves. Mothers were in deep distress over missing children.

I wondered what would happen to me if I were ever in such a disaster. Would I be left behind because of my disability? I thought of the elderly abandoned to die, and remembered Mama and Daddy in their closing years when they were both dependent on others. I tried to imagine the sheer terror that someone's mom or dad must have felt as they watched the water rising, knowing no one would save them. In preparing for my recent surgery, I was advised to have an Advanced Care Directive. Had I been in a hospital in New Orleans during the hurricane, would that have mattered? I had been on a ventilator for four days. Would I have been considered worth saving?

I do not pretend to understand this depth of anguish or why God allows it. I only know that God is good and promised to one day put an end to all suffering. This is the truth that sustains me and causes joy to thrive even in the midst of grief.

## A TALE OF TWO TITTIES

"It was the best of times, it was the worst of times..." Teetee and Boobie were twins, though not identical. Teetee was bigger and remained so throughout their natural lives. These girls were very close as they grew up sharing the carefree days of early childhood. They remained close during their teenage years, when together they endured the embarrassment of crude men's digs. Their companionship continued strong even through years of childbearing and nursing.

One day, a terrible thing happened and Boobie was taken away, never to be seen again. How Teetee mourned her loss! Though she had a family, she could not endure the loss of her twin. So she headed south in search of a new buddy.

Several years later, Teetee heard that a companion had been found; she allowed herself to be brought back from down south. Imagine her joy when Teetee met her new friend. She looked almost like Boobie. She felt warm and alive. Teetee was thrilled! She had been so lonely! She knew it wasn't Boobie, but it was as close as she would ever get to having a bosom buddy again.

Teetee's contentment with her new companion is often ruffled by the thought that what happened to Boobie could someday happen to her too. When these thoughts invade, she thrusts them aside, trusting God that it will not be so. For now, she will enjoy her new companion and revel in the gifts that each day brings. 2005

## NO PAIN NO GAIN

Often wishing she had not
Of boobs and belly such a lot,
When cancer took away her breast,
She placed her belly on her chest.

When Doc her tummy from her took
He gave to her a tummy tuck.
Now her apple shape is gone,
Her risk for heart disease gone down.

Two smaller boobs are here to stay,
Prosthesis and girdles thrown away.
In spite of all the fear and pain,
From cancer she's derived great gain.

Breast reconstruction was implemented in several phases. I chose the DIEP flap surgery (deep inferior epigastric perforators). A flap of tissue with blood vessels, skin and fat from my lower abdomen was transferred to my chest. The surgeon attached the blood vessels of the flap to the blood vessels of my chest. He then formed a new breast that looked natural, and, with my belly rerouted, I looked slimmer. Initially, I experienced severe pain and abdominal weakness, which improved over time.

Before the second phase, I experienced bouts of nausea and vomiting. In January 2006, I was back in the hospital for gallbladder surgery. In phase 2, adjustments were done on the reconstructed breast and the left was downsized to match.

A few weeks later, I developed an infection in my left breast and was again hospitalized. Thinking I had recovered sufficiently, I returned to the gym. My right breast was still bandaged, but I felt great.

One day, after returning from the gym, I was changing the bandage and found, to my horror, that my breast was split open. I sobbed in dismay, thinking the surgery was ruined. When I called the surgeon crying, he casually told me to come see him. "Doc" put me back together again and the healing proceeded without further alarm.

The first attempt to create a nipple flunked; it went flat after healing. We tried again, this time in the doctor's office. He used tissue from my thigh to form the nipple. When this attempt failed, I should have returned for another try. One day I thought, "Better leave well enough alone," and never went back. I'm not completely symmetrical, but who is? These days, I live like a normal woman, not having to think about cancer every time I dress. What freedom!

## *TRANSITION*

I have been a divorced, single, stay-at-home mom,
And have watched son and daughter dress up for their prom.
Though they've flown the coop in search of new fodder,
I am, by no means, an unhappy mother.
I'm enjoying this time of tranquility
While staving off the approach of senility.

There is food in the fridge and the dishes are clean.
It's so blessedly still and I don't want to scream.
The computer is not tied up, the telephone rings
And I can actually find all my things.
The messes I clean up are now all my own
And no one complains if I sleep-talk or moan.

I am now seeking a new enterprise
And am willing to try on suggestions for size.
I need to pursue some new interesting thing
Or find me a beau and have me a fling.
But I'm so enjoying my new solitude,
I will not give it up for just any old dude.

If I had more than just nickels and dimes,
I think I'd be traveling much of the time.
That it would be more fun with someone by my side
Is an obvious truth I am not going to hide.
That a man with much dough and a very good eye
Would fulfill such a need, I will never deny.

I would like a new friend, but don't want to lose me.
Is there a good man who could let me be free
To be myself and not try to control?
Could he be himself without strangling my soul?
Should I take the risk with the hope I might find
A gentleman and a true valentine?

# JOY IN REFLECTION

Dear Daughter,

I've watched you from a baby, strong-willed, determined to acquire whatever your heart desired. As your mother, I've been challenged to direct those desires toward good things. You asked me once when you were small, "Does being strong-willed mean I'm bad?" I replied, "Oh no!" It was from God you got that will, determination to succeed in the face of opposition. It means that you can conquer anything to which you set your mind. When you establish a goal, you will pursue it to its finish.

I knew your will, bent towards God, would accomplish much good. The challenge of being your mom made me strong! I had to dig in my heels to steer you away from wrong.

I've watched you struggle through the divorce and wounds inflicted by rejection. I've watched you yearning for your Daddy's love. You often asked, "Mom, should I call again?" I always said it was your choice, and supported you in your resolve to protect your heart from further wounding.

Despite our power struggles, you did demonstrate your caring and insight, as expressed in the following letter you wrote to me during your junior high years. It moved me to tears, realizing that you understood so much at such a tender age. A mother could desire no greater tribute.

"Dear Mommy,

I am writing this to thank you for all you have done for me. Thank you for the sacrifices you have made so that I could be able to attend a Christian school. The one year that I went to public school, I had a very hard time with the atmosphere. Everything had to be so politically correct, to the point that you could hardly speak about anything. When I started attending school here in sixth grade, it made me very happy. I knew all about the money you had to spend on uniforms, and field trips, and tuition. I'm sure that at times you did not know where the money would come from. However, I never had to worry about money or transportation or anything. Also, thank you for homeschooling me. Many people do not understand how much work and sacrifice goes into homeschooling your children. Especially when you are a single parent, and have to live with a disability. Without homeschooling, I would not be the person I am today. Lastly, thank you for being my mother. Thank you for all you have done to raise me and make me into a woman after God's own heart. I may not be the model child, but I'm well on my way.

I love you very much,

Agalia"

God providentially placed you in Mrs. Gee's sixth grade class. She had lost her mom at age 13 and was very aware of your emotional conflict as you watched me battle cancer. You always shared with me the supportive comments she wrote in your journal. I have known Mrs. Gee for more than 30 years and we have a tight bond. For several years, I have enjoyed volunteering in her classroom, sharing poetry and giving presentations on Jamaica and visual impairment.

I watched you struggle in high school and recall the tears and panic, your difficulty going out the door. It was a time when you were so unsure. I remember being afraid that you might fail. In the end, you bolstered your will to finish well. Finding the way yourself, you graduated six months early.

Evangelism Explosion was your call. You were pursuing matters of eternal value. I was so pleased when you received your commendation. Your sensitivity towards good made me lift my praise to God. You showed caring for the neighbor kids, desiring that they should know your God. I remember the Bible you bought for

Marcus when he joined the military and the hours you spent challenging him.

When Grandma sent us food, you were always quick to share. You would have given it all away, had I not intervened. I watched your love for kids emerge as you cared for Sonya's twins. You baked cookies with the neighbors and played with Elena's hair, perhaps yearning for a little sister. Babysitting and childcare are some of your strongest assets. You've shown much empathy for the underdog, often telling me stories of people not treated fairly. Tiny tots in daycare crying for their mommies always touched a chord in you.

I beamed inside as your grades soared during your freshman year at U.S. Center for World Missions. You were in your element. The social butterfly had found her garden. On the phone, your joy effervesced into giggles in a room filled with high-spirited girls. Your friends were people of whom I could be proud. Your strong will and faith were winning.

It was your choice to become a vegetarian and you never swayed despite criticism or ribbing. It was also your choice when you decided to give it up. I've watched you learn to shop for and cook the food you chose to eat. I love your cooking and Grandma does too.

You embarked on another course when you applied to college. God has a plan for you that's not yet seen. It was no surprise when, on Missions Sunday, you responded to the call of God. I had seen your bent, your strong intent to do His will. God is molding you. The process is not painless, but neither is it joyless.

I know, in spite of growing pains, that you will stay the course. I wait with eagerness to see God's woman emerge from her cocoon. I anticipate the brilliance that will impact the world from this gem God is right now polishing. Already I glimpse a sparkle of things to come and joyfully anticipate the rewards of my labor.

I wish you spiritual maturity in choosing the father of my grandchildren. I wish you a healthy baby machine! I'm staying alive for that, girl! I wish you scholarships to help you through school and many more years of joy! Happy 20th Birthday!

Mom

Lord Jesus, thank You for the beautiful daughter with whom You chose to bless me. You loaned her to me, so now that she's a woman, I release her into Your care and into the care of others You will bring into her life. Transform her into the image of Jesus. Free her from bitterness. Let Your pure unselfish love rule her life and guard her heart. May trials make her strong and even more determined to go on, walking in step with You.

Enable her to look within and acknowledge the things that need changing. Grant me the joy of seeing her grow to maturity in You. Pour out Your favor on her and give her evidence that You are indeed her Heavenly Father, able and willing to do more than she can imagine. Give her the desires of her heart as they increasingly reflect Your desires. Thank you for the privilege of being her mother and the ultimate privilege of leading her into a relationship with You.

## APPLES OF GOLD

I met Julie in the setting of a Silver Saturday celebration. As the guest speaker, she introduced herself as a two-time breast cancer survivor and a journalism professor. When she mentioned the class "Writing for Wellness," I knew I had to meet her.

As I introduced myself, her inviting words were like "apples of gold" and have continued to be just that for me and so many others. I began attending Julie's journalism classes and later joined the Writing for Wellness class she started at City of Hope after September 11th, 2001. She has motivated me to pursue other forms of writing in addition to poetry, and my self-confidence as a writer has grown.

This class remained a source of support and enrichment for several years. Julie made everyone comfortable. It was a pleasure to watch people grow in confidence and skill, after initially declaring their inability to write. I relished the opportunity to share my writing in an atmosphere of acceptance, and the encouragement derived from hearing other survivor stories. The experience was therapeutic. Our class was filmed by both ABC and CBS News. On one of those occasions, I appeared on the evening news, sharing a portion of the poem "So What I Have No Valentine!"

A member of our class, James Cremin (now deceased), filmed a documentary where I can be heard singing "Mastectomy Song" and playing background music on the piano.

Julie was generous and genuinely caring. Her willingness to share her skills and talents with us was praiseworthy. The loving care poured into the culinary repasts with which she delighted us each time we met, reminded me of Mama.

Julie inspired me to take one of the biggest steps since cancer— my *breastoration*. "A Tale of Two Titties" would never have been written without her influence. I recall many rides home and her concern for me during tough times.

In 2007, thanks to Julie's vision and expertise, *Writing for Wellness: A Prescription for Healing* was published. It is a compilation of contributions from cancer survivors and caregivers. We all agreed that the proceeds from the book would be donated to the City of Hope to aid in ongoing cancer research. It was our way of giving back. With the help of this book, several similar classes have been started elsewhere. The day I met Julie, I couldn't have imagined such a remarkable outcome.

Julie, I hope you are around for a long time and continue to be the special person you are. In your silver years, may your words continue to be apples of gold (Proverbs 25:11).

## *I SAW CHRISTINE TODAY*

I barely glimpsed her silhouetted form
Through the window of her bone marrow ward.
I could not see the covering on her head,
The pallor of her skin or eyes,
Or the fragility of her weakened body.
But I saw Christine today.
I looked into the window of her soul
And clearly saw her gentle spirit.

Her serenity and strength were evident.
I heard and felt her smiles and tears
As she read aloud with keen appreciation
The prayer I had written for her.

The rhythmic cadence of her voice
Made me momentarily forget
That here was a woman fighting for her life.
We gazed into each other's souls with wonder.
It was an electrifying connection of two kindred spirits
Who have known adversity and the triumph of faith.
My eyes could not look into Christine's eyes,
But I clearly saw into her soul today.
I cannot read the mind of God
Regarding Christine's future,
But I know here is a soul,
A being refined through suffering. 2006

Christine Pechera survived Non-Hodgkin's lymphoma after two bone marrow transplants. In searching for her own donor, she saved other lives by increasing awareness of the need for volunteers to register as potential donors (especially from minorities) in the National Marrow Donor Program (Be The Match)."

Aware of the disparity in diagnosis and treatment of cancer among minorities, the Center of Community Alliance for Research & Education (CCARE) at City of Hope Medical Center in California, has instituted the Annual Minority Cancer Awareness Week Forum. Researchers, medical professionals, community advocates, and cancer survivors interact to address these disparities. I have been invited for several years to close the forum with the following poem.

## TOGETHER WE STAND

"Two heads are better than one," we have heard
And two hearts care better than one is inferred.
We are gathered here to join heads and hearts
For those whose lives cancer is ripping apart.

From our dialoguing today,
Some pearls of wisdom may open the way
To research that could, in the end, find a cure
Or at least make life better for others, I'm sure.

Let's roll up our sleeves, don our thinking caps;
Each one may provide what the other lacks.
Let's listen and hear the concerns of each other,
For the community needs what researchers offer.

We must foster mutual trust and respect
For community and researchers to interact.
Then together we'll stand with one common aim—
We will stand up to cancer and end all this pain! 2008

## I WON

The "disease to please" had been "killing me softly."
Rejection plunged my immunity into a downward spiral.
When Mama died, something in me died too.
Then cancer seized the day,
Spreading its toxic tentacles through my pain-riddled breast.
The lump appeared, sounding its ominous death knell,
Shocking me out of my self-pitying stupor,
Propelling me to life-affirming action.
Aiming my prayers heavenward to muster faith and courage,
I seized the day!
Reclaiming my personal power, I fought for hope,
For healing and joy in living—I won! 2007 (11-year anniversary)

# UNFORGETTABLE

On December 1st, 2006, I received the Section 8 voucher for which I had waited 15 years. The voucher entitled me to a rental subsidy. I had placed my name on a waiting list shortly after the separation. Although my landlord had said he wouldn't accept it, I asked again.

"Would you do it for just one year? I would have time to save money for moving."

"No! I don't like doing business with those people." Voucher recipients had 60 days to find a place. Only one extension of another 60 days could be granted. Agalia was working abroad but would live with me when she returned. The case worker crossed her name off the application, saying it could be added later. The new rule was one bedroom for two people. The idea of sharing a bedroom with my young adult daughter did not seem feasible, but what were my options?

A friend told me of an available rental close to church; it was upstairs in back of a larger house. The rent was less than the Housing Authority allowed for a single bedroom. While looking over the place, my type "A" brain mentally placed furniture, wondering how we would fit. I was cringing at the potential stress. "Lord," I prayed, "I will make whatever sacrifice You want me to make, but this is going to be hard." The landlady was willing to consider Section 8, so I filled out the application.

My OCD brain would not let me sleep that night. I tried, but kept getting up to pack a few more things as I organized the process in my head. I had regularly discarded unwanted items. This time, I was sorting through things with a fine-tooth comb. It's interesting how boxes multiply when you are packing to move. Things that don't look like much on a shelf seem to be so much more when packed in boxes. I had emptied the closets of everything except my clothing. Pictures were cleared from the walls. Knickknacks, bedding, most of the kitchen items, books and Agalia's belongings had been boxed when I received an early morning call from my landlord.

"I've been thinking and I changed my mind. I will accept the voucher."

"Are you serious? I already packed up most of the apartment."

"I realize it is going to be very hard for you to find a place and you have been through so much. My wife thinks I should keep you because you have been here so long and have been a good tenant." Surprised, I momentarily mused, my emotions conflicted.

"Well, I am still waiting for a call on another apartment I checked out. I will get back to you when I hear something." Within an hour the call came; that apartment had been rented. I knew God had changed my landlord's heart. Happy at the news, my neighbor, Casandra, offered to help me put the apartment back together to give the inspector a good impression. Essentially, he would be checking to make sure the landlord had everything in working order.

I groaned from exhaustion, looking at the mountain of boxes. I had groaned even more at the thought of moving everything in my apartment down those steep stairs, across town and up some more stairs. My last move had been 23 years earlier and only from next door. Unpacking was more physically exhausting than it was emotional. There had been an underlying peace that God would grant the desire of my heart.

After Agalia went overseas, I discarded her bed; it was in bad shape, having been dragged from dorm to house-sharing and back home. I planned to replace the bed before her return. In light of the anticipated inspection, I decided to do it right away. The rent was within the allowed limits for a single bedroom, so the extra room would not be an issue. Shortly after realizing I would not have to move, I received a long-distance phone call.

Agalia was working as a nanny and tutor, but the challenge had proven overwhelming and she was coming home sooner than expected. Good thing I had bought her a new bed. No decision was wasted. She arrived the day before inspection.

"I may have to hide you. I just want the inspection to go smoothly, then I can deal with the fact that you are back and how it will impact everything."

"Tell them I just came back. Can't someone stay with you for a few weeks before you have to report it?"

Despite my quandary, I passed the inspection. God is good! I breathed a sigh of relief. It was done. The pressure was off. My rent would be substantially reduced, and there wouldn't be another inspection until the next year.

"Taste and see that the Lord is good; blessed is the man who takes refuge in him." Psalm 34:8

## JOY REKINDLED

Dear Son,

Times were hard for us after your father left. My dreams for our family were shattered. God hates divorce because of the emotional violence it inflicts on those involved. Crazed with pain, I tried to do my best for you and your sister, though it was a job meant for two. Often feeling like a failure, I begged God to protect you from my blunders.

The odds were against me as I struggled by myself to give you a good life. Believe me, it was hard being a single mother. I was often flying by the seat of my pants. Parenting under the best circumstances is difficult and I am far from perfect. Please forgive me for any injury I caused you unwittingly in my own frustration.

As you approached adolescence, you began challenging my authority. Warning about the danger for a young Black boy walking the streets after hours, I tried to hold the reins so you wouldn't self-destruct. One night, I emerged from a deep sleep, wondering if I had made the right decision. I had given you permission for a sleep-over at your friend's house. You failed to mention a party elsewhere. The pain and guilt following that disturbing phone call was indescribable. If only I hadn't said yes. I could have lost you!

Your "testosterone-driven madness" coincided with Grandpa's illness and death. You were clearly out of control. I had to take a tough love stand, the hardest thing I have ever done. My motivation was to protect you by setting limits. Dr. James Dobson wrote a book called *Parenting is Not for Cowards*. I think you will understand that best when you become a parent.

You gave me the cold shoulder for a while, but wanting to show how much I still loved you, I brought you your 18th birthday gift. It was another in the *Left Behind* series by Tim Lahaye. You always enjoyed his books. I prayed for you real hard, and many people assured me that you would be back.

"He's a good boy," someone encouraged. "He's struggling with separating from you but he'll be back. When there is a divorce, kids always give the parent who stays the hardest time; it's because they feel safer with you."

I was pleased when you returned home at my invitation. You wanted to be independent and came with a plan. You exhibited good work ethics and I had no worry in that regard. Sometimes I got up to see if you were awake, but you had already left for work.

I recall with pleasure the Valentine's Day when you burst in the door during your work break to bring me a beautiful freesia plant. I will always remember with fondness my birthday and Mother's Day dinners at various venues. Your invitation to me and my girlfriends to celebrate my 60th birthday was precious. You gave us a memorable evening. The ladies were impressed and I felt very special. That fig martini you made me was my first. What a treat!

At the Red Gem, we created a memory that will forever cause me to smile. The sound of your strong masculine voice and laughter, the exquisite tastes and pungent aromas of the dishes we sampled, and the joy these evoked from my friends, will be cherished memories. Thank you for giving Don a wonderful 74th birthday. He and Margie are always willing to transport us to and from the airport, and have treated Agalia and me to many birthday dinners.

You have found your niche in life and pursue your goals with passion. You are such an extrovert! The restaurant business definitely suits you. Your coworkers adored you. No wonder the owner didn't want you to leave. It must be great to know you have options. That is a good place to be. You earned it!

I like to think I taught you everything you know; the truth is, I lit the fire, and you have carried the torch. You are an industrious and independent young man. The result of your hard work and commitment is evident. I thank God for giving me a wonderful son and continue to pray His blessings on you in all your endeavors. You make me proud!

Your vest from Awana Cubbies reminds me that, even as a child, you knew the Scriptures that lead to salvation. I pray that your walk with God will be renewed. I pray that your life will be pleasing to Him in every way. May He send you a godly wife and grant you a successful marriage. I especially pray for my grandkids. I want my turn to sit back and laugh at you, as you tell them some of the same things I told you. You think you won't? Just wait and see!

I am so glad God gave, or rather loaned, you to me. His hand has been on your life since before you were born and will continue to be there until the day you die. You and I share DNA. You are bone of my bones and flesh of my flesh. You are my son and that will never change. I love you deeply and that will never change. I am here for you and I wish I could say that will never change. The fact is, life is brief and tomorrow is not promised; however, as long as I am here, my heart and my arms are open to you. While the going is good, let's make some new memories. Happy 26th Birthday!

Mom

"You turned my wailing into dancing; you removed my sackcloth and clothed me with joy." Psalm 30:11

# MY PERSONAL EARTHQUAKE

The rumbling began as I walked into the gym one morning. A dull pain in my left side persisted through water aerobics. Uncomfortable all day, I kept massaging my side hoping for some relief. About 8:30 that night, the discomfort intensified. As I was describing it to the nurse on the phone, the pain suddenly quadrupled in intensity. I writhed in agony. A wave of nausea swept over me as pain radiated through my abdomen and lower back.

I sobbed as paramedics carried me down the stairs. One of the EMT's remembered being at my house the month before, responding to an asthma attack. I thought to myself, "I just turned 60 and this is already the second time I have called 9-1-1. Is a pattern developing here?"

I alternated between whimpering and wailing, and calling for the Lord Jesus as the ER staff performed the preliminaries. My left side felt as if it was in a vise. I swallowed some pain medication, then threw up. Technicians whisked me away for an X-ray. I threw up again.

"How intense is the pain on a scale from 1-10?"

"Ten," I moaned without hesitation. It was more like 20 on my personal Richter scale. I suffered severe dysmenorrheal cramps back in the day, but this was different. When I received morphine intravenously, my hand began to burn. More pain, just what I needed! Without warning, projectile vomiting dislodged the remains of my dinner, leaving a bilious taste in my mouth. The abdominal paroxysms increased. Deciding the medicine was too strong, the doctor gave me Zofran, good old Zofran! It had rescued me during chemo. My pain had subsided to about five, and I was half asleep when the doctor woke me up.

"We're sending you home."

"What do you mean you're sending me home? You haven't given me an explanation for this pain. I'm not going home like this."

"Well, the X-ray doesn't show anything."

I argued with him until he called my HMO. Thank God! He received authorization to admit me. My potassium was low. I was transferred to the observation unit with a heart monitor, and remained there until late afternoon on Wednesday. A CT scan was ordered, and I was moved to another room. I received a huge container of a bland-tasting liquid, the only thing that had passed my lips since dinner on Tuesday.

After the scan, I was served a meal and wolfed it down. Soon the pain began to escalate again. I requested morphine with Zofran and had a restful night.

While I was in the hospital, my "Writing for Wellness" class at City of Hope was being filmed for another documentary. Although disappointed, I took it in stride. On Thursday morning, the nurse announced my discharge. I hadn't heard from the doctor and insisted on waiting for him. He never showed. I returned home, still sore and clueless regarding the cause of the pain. 2008

## SIXTY YEARS TODAY

Sixty years today,
Still no wrinkles or laugh lines,
Just good genetics.
Sixty years today,
Now hips and knees are creaking.
Body betrays me.
Sixty years today,
Positive outlook on life,
Spirit is at peace.
Sixty years today,
Looking forward to much more.
God's not done with me. 2008

## THE AFTERNOON I FLEW
(Tune: "Ode to Joy" or "I've Been Working on The Railroad")

I was standing on my step-stool
With my arms up in the air,
As I opened up a cupboard
To replace some items there.

Then a crack and jerk beneath me
Suddenly filled my heart with dread.
I knew I was going to fall,
And perhaps upon my head.

In a moment I was airborne,
Arms were flailing left and right.
I was actually flying!
Oh, it must have been a sight!
Then, five feet away I landed
Hard upon my derriere,
Missing tabletop and counter,
Even a few scattered chairs.

I was stunned, I have to tell you,
But I lived to tell the tale.
Were it not for Silver Sneakers,
My neighbors would have heard me wail.
But instead, I groaned a little,
Picked myself up off the floor,
Looked down at my broken step-stool,
Then resumed my household chores.

Secure Horizons' Silver Sneakers,
You have made me strong, 'tis true!
And I never will forget you
Nor the afternoon I flew.
You must never end this program.
Who knows what I might do next?
Keep it coming, Silver Sneakers,
Secure Horizons, you're the best!

Silver Sneakers, yes!
The more of you, the less of stress,
The more of you, of me the less,
Secure Horizons, you're the best!  2009

## GYM CAROL
(Tune: "Have Yourself a Merry Little Christmas")

Have yourselves a diet-conscious Christmas!
May your weight be light!
From now on the scales will all be out of sight.
It's the time of year we wreck our diets,
Gaining many pounds.
Don't forget those pounds they like to stick around.
Anything placed between the lips will upon the hips remain.
Just remember that losing weight can be such a pain!
Don't forget to count your carbohydrates as you eat your food.
Santa's watching you to see if you are good.
Then next year we will all be here
And we'll know how much you've gained.
Instructors dear also will be here
And they'll be causing us much pain!
So have yourselves a merry little Christmas!
Don't eat like a sow!
Hang that pumpkin pie upon the highest bough,
And have yourselves a diet-conscious Christmas now! 2009

## JOY IN JAMAICA AGAIN

The night before this trip, I was again in the emergency room, experiencing low-grade abdominal cramping. The discomfort had become more unbearable as bedtime approached. Knowing I would be sitting on the airplane for a long time, I had thought it best to call 9-1-1.

Diverticulitis was the diagnosis. I was advised to avoid nuts, but a bag of almonds was already stashed in my suitcase. The doctor suggested I postpone the trip; I could end up in the hospital in Jamaica. How could I cancel? I was going to a wedding. After procuring some pain medication, I took my chances.

At the airport, security pulled me aside. Someone questioned me about gunpowder residue detected in the wheelchair I was using. The chair belonged to the airport, but I was suspect. While I waited, several uniformed men huddled in private conference a few feet from me. My innocence was eventually confirmed, and I was free to continue my journey.

Jamaica was unseasonably cool when I arrived. It rained heavily that Friday evening, but cleared up for the wedding on Saturday. Ghana, the bride, was elegantly dressed in a beaded, sleeveless, ankle-length white dress without a veil or train. Her dreadlocks were woven into a beehive on top of her head and studded with white beads. Shari, Ghana's sister and maid of honor, wearing dark brown, carried a bouquet of orange flowers, while the bridesmaids sported orange dresses and family members, all in dreadlocks, wore varying shades of brown.

In 2009, after being diagnosed with pre-diabetes, I lost 30 lbs. A fashionable, form-fitting cocoa brown dress trimmed with beige embroidery was my reward. It was purchased months before I knew there would be a wedding.

During the ceremony, the groom's mother stood by her son, Roberto, singing. Mardell, the bride's mother, joined her. It was an emotional moment when the mothers' voices broke and tears of joy flowed. An informal reception was held in a white tent on the church lawn, beneath swaying palm trees. Following toasts to the new couple, and the cutting of the cake, family and close friends moved to the Hilton for an afternoon lunch. I was privileged to share a poem dedicated to the happy couple.

A few days after the wedding, the 2010 Haiti earthquake shook Jamaica. Although tsunami alerts warned against going near the water, days later, boatloads of Haitian refugees reached our shores.

Auntie Joy was delighted to meet many cousins, old and young, especially the little ones, who reveled in the gifts they received. Although she had not lived to see them, Grace now had four grandchildren. I met my great-nephews for the first time. Her two granddaughters would be moving to Jamaica from Japan and I looked forward to meeting them on my next visit. Moving from house to house, I ate delicious food and reconnected with old acquaintances, including my high school headmistress, who was 90 years old.

Before my departure, I was a guest at the National Leadership Prayer Breakfast. In attendance were the Governor General, Prime Minister, Leader of the Opposition, judicial and church leaders. Jamaica was a troubled country. The murder rate hit a record high in 2009—16,803 murders in just one year, compared to 30,000 murders for the previous decade. The nation was called to return to Biblical values. Earnest prayer went up for the state of the country and the people who were hurting. Taxation was also very high. The dollar exchange was then 89 Jamaican dollars to $1 USD. Everything, including food, was taxed at 17.5%. Imagine paying several thousand dollars to fill your gas tank!

Jamaica was still beautiful in spite of the hardships, and I enjoyed reconnecting with my roots. Freedom from paperwork and a chattering computer for two whole weeks was an added bonus.

# PROVIDENTIAL PROVISION

"Your landlord has raised the rent, so the amount you pay after the subsidy will be $200 more. Why don't you talk to him? You have been a long-time tenant; perhaps he will agree not to raise it." The landlord agreed to freeze the rent temporarily, but, according to the housing authorities, Agalia, who would soon graduate from college, would no longer be able to live with me. It was time to find a senior apartment.

At the beginning of 2011, I started downsizing, packing and labeling boxes in Braille and print, and setting items aside for a yard sale. Compiling a list of senior apartments, I began the hunt. At 63, life was not over, and living in a claustrophobic box would not be acceptable. I needed a home with room to invite a friend or two for dinner, as well as space for an office. I was losing heart after a yearlong, fruitless search, when Avizi called.

"Hi Mom, you won't believe this! I was chatting with a customer who wanted to know where I was from. When I told him, he asked how I liked the city. I said, 'It's cool!' Then he responded, 'Well, I'm glad you said that because I am the Mayor!' "

"Really? How interesting!" I laughed.

"We chatted some more, and before he left, he handed me his card and told me to give it to you. He wants you to call him if you ever have any problems."

"Wow! I will definitely call him. Maybe he can help me find senior housing here."

I had lived in the same city for 32 years and I preferred to stay there if possible. The Mayor was a man of his word. Two days after I called him, a social worker visited me with a list of available apartments. The second listing surprised me. I had passed the place for years, never suspecting it held senior housing.

Although the building and its location were impressive, my heart sank when I saw the size of the one bedroom. It was definitely too small. On returning home, I called my sister who worked for a senior housing program. She suggested I submit a request for reasonable accommodation. A letter from my doctor helped seal the deal.

On seeing the new apartment, I exclaimed with relief, "Yes, I can do this!" It was way better than I had anticipated. There were two bedrooms and two bathrooms. A sliding door opened unto a balcony from the living area. No claustrophobia here! The smaller bedroom was the perfect size for my office furniture. Never having had the luxury of a dishwasher or garbage disposal, I especially loved the kitchen. There was a trash chute just a little way from my door and a laundry room on the way from the elevator. Everything I would need was right there.

The following Sunday, I received an envelope with a Christmas gift from my church. I was grateful, of course, but was not yet aware of its significance. On Monday, I called the apartment manager.

"I love that apartment! Please don't give it to anyone else. I have an appointment with Housing to pick up my voucher on January 4th."

"I can't hold it too long," said the manager, "but if you can give me a deposit, I will reserve it for 30 days." The deposit was exactly the amount of the gift I had just received. This was clearly God at work. I was in awe! Meanwhile, my lower back problems had worsened. I was in constant pain. The day before the big move, I had a second epidural and was not in the best shape. I would be "moving on up" to the fifth floor, but thank God, via elevator!

While things were falling into place for me, Agalia, who had graduated from college in May, was getting anxious. It was the middle of December. She had started a full-time job just two weeks earlier. Needing to find an apartment and a roommate, she wondered if it would all happen in time.

On January 20th, 2012, Avizi and a crew of friends took charge. I was in my new home by noon. Exhausted, yet elated, I reveled in the fact that God had again provided beyond my wildest expectations.

"How great is your goodness which you have stored up for those who fear you, which you bestow in the sight of men on those who take refuge in you. Psalm 31:19

February 7, 2012

Even after two weeks, I still can't believe this is all mine. I feel so blessed. This week, with Ellen's help, I put Braille labels on the dishwasher and microwave, and hung pictures. Thanks to my internet provider, I have been off-line for two weeks. Last night, I cried myself to sleep after spending six hours on the phone with customer service. I was trying to set up email. There's always something threatening to steal my joy. Nevertheless, I am thrilled and grateful to all who helped with the move.

God's timing is perfect! Agalia met a roommate online mid-January, and on January 16th, they found a place. Two days later, my daughter contacted the manager, who requested that she bring in her application the following day. Agalia explained that she worked all day and didn't drive. Believe it or not, the manager, a complete stranger, went to her job to collect the application. Someone had applied before them. I prayed that God would remove all obstacles. Agalia moved into her new apartment on January 28th. We had until the 31st to vacate the old premises. What a mighty God we serve! The blessings keep coming! Avizi was promoted to manager at the restaurant where he works. There is nothing more pleasing to a mom than to see her children doing well.

February 27, 2012

Another attack of diverticulitis landed me in the hospital. The intense pain was eventually alleviated by medication delivered intravenously. There is an upside to this. I worked very hard all last year, preparing to move, moving, and unpacking. While in the hospital, my meals were catered, although just Jell-O, clear broth and tea; someone was constantly checking on me; I even had my back and feet rubbed with lotion. When was the last time that happened?

Once the pain was under control, I saw this episode as a mini-vacation and pampering I wouldn't have had otherwise. Well, pampering is over. I am home, and if I don't work, I don't eat.

"The Lord is good, a refuge in times of trouble. He cares for those who trust in him." Nahum 1:7

## *JOY ENTERS THE HOUSE*

Before you were born,
I asked God for a daughter.
He sent you to me.
"Joy enters the house!"
That's the meaning of your name.
Your birth brought great joy,
Then, for a season,
Trials tried to stifle joy,
But God heard my cries.
Through the ups and downs
Of life's uncertain promise,
Jesus buoyed us up.

I would like to say
That I taught you all you know,
But that's so not true!
The Master Teacher,
Granting you a fertile mind,
Planted wisdom there.
With much toil and care,
Your beauty now has blossomed
Into womanhood.
And I am so proud,
So proud to call you daughter!
Congratulations!

Agalia's graduation from college, May 5, 2011

"May he give you the desires of your heart and make all your plans succeed. We will shout for joy when you are victorious and will lift up our banners in the name of our God." Psalm 20:4, 5

## LIVING AS A VIP

I am a VIP and I know it! Do I sound conceited? Well, it depends on how you *see* it. Being a VIP (visually impaired person) places me in the category of having special needs rather than special privileges. Though not completely blind, I have lost enough vision to make it impossible to function in a visual world without special adaptations.

There is a continuum from fully sighted to fully blind. A person can be parked anywhere along that continuum. In my case, I am more than halfway to the blind side, not parked, but moving slowly. Being partially sighted is quite different from being completely blind, and therefore has its peculiar problems. The average sighted person is often unsure of how to respond to the confusion of a progressive loss of vision. Living as a VIP is hard enough. The way others respond can facilitate or make it more burdensome.

While struggling with my new reality, I actually encountered people who thought I was faking it. Other overly solicitous souls presumed to know what kind of help I needed without asking. One day I was standing on a street corner. A man, spotting the white cane, promptly lifted my cane-carrying arm up in the air and dragged me across the street. He then bothered to ask where I was going. "I am meeting someone here," I replied, obviously annoyed. The questions "May I help?" or "How can I help?" would have clarified the situation.

One day, a woman and a little girl were walking my way. The youngster asked, "Why do you have that stick?" The mother immediately pulled her back, apologizing.

"It's okay," I said. "The way to get answers is to ask questions." I explained to the child that I can't see everything that she sees, then demonstrated how the cane helps me.

Another day, as I walked down the street, minding my own business, a man shouted, "Get rid of that stick! You don't need it!" I think he needed *that stick* over his head for being so rude. A Good Samaritan, doing his good deed for the day, hoisted me on to the bus and paid my fare. Fingering the free bus pass in my pocket, I stifled a chuckle. A "significant other" (no longer significant) often insisted that I fold up my white cane. He then watched me walk into the cement blocks in the parking lot or trip on unfamiliar stairs before coming to my aid.

When I first learned to use the white cane, I was very self-conscious and often wished I could do without it. I sometimes tried to "pass" as a sighted person. One day, I walked to a nearby store without the cane. I had to cross a very busy street and I managed. Coming back was daunting. The stream of traffic seemed unending. Just then, a woman approached the crosswalk. Plucking up my courage, I asked for help, explaining that I was legally blind and had left my cane at home. She promptly scolded me.

"Why don't you have your cane? The cane is what helps motorists know that you can't see. Don't you ever do that again!" Accepting that the white cane alerts others to my disability, I have never done that again. Kind pedestrians have frequently steered me clear of obstacles because they saw the cane.

Although I've lost my central vision, I still have some peripheral vision. I am uncomfortable and don't mingle well in a room full of people, strangers or not. I will never see my "true love across a crowded room." If I look directly at a person in front of me, I do not see their face and cannot read their expression. If I try to look in a way that I can see (sideways), I sometimes see a stranger squirm with discomfort, probably wondering why I am avoiding eye contact.

"When I first met you, you wouldn't look at me. I thought you didn't like me because my English was not good." Kiem, an Indonesian friend, told me this after we had known each other for a long time. I'm not an unfriendly person, yet I've often been called a snob for failing to make eye contact.

I was standing in the checkout line at a store; my friend stepped away for a minute. The clerk was handing me the receipt when Pamela returned. She placed my hand on the line for my signature. The clerk blurted out, "Oh my G...! I thought I was ugly and that's why you wouldn't look at me. I didn't know you couldn't see!" Her reaction was over the top! I smiled, but when we left the store, Pamela and I couldn't stop laughing.

Although I try to *look good,* I'm never sure how my *good looks* will affect people. Once, while teaching a backyard Bible class, I tried to stare down an unruly kid, hoping he would stop misbehaving. I could see (from my peripheral vision) several kids squirming in discomfort, while the offender remained oblivious.

I purchased my first computer in 1998. My initial project was to transfer 200 poems to Microsoft Word. It was a thrill being able to make corrections without having to start from scratch, as I did in the days of the typewriter. I have upgraded computers several times and now use Windows 7. Each upgrade presents a steep learning curve. Why do people fix things that aren't broken?

To access the computer, I use a screen reader called JAWS (job acquisition with speech). The constant monotonous drone of this electronic voice is like a hammer at the side of my head. Sometimes I scream in frustration, "Shut up!" Good thing the voice doesn't respond to audible commands. I wouldn't get anything done. Sometimes a dialog box pops up; I can see it, but can't read it, and JAWS is not responding. I may have to restart the computer or abandon the task until a sighted person is available. Navigating the web is most frustrating! Many websites are not user-friendly for a screen reader user. Sighted helpers are annoyed with JAWS. They can turn it off and continue working. I don't have that option.

"Open Book" is a speech software that utilizes a scanner. A printed page is placed on the scanner; the command is given via keystrokes; the print is read audibly; the document can then be edited. Adaptive technology has revolutionized my life; yet it is so expensive, you need a job to afford it, but can't get a job without it.

The CCTV was upgraded after 20 years; however, its functionality has decreased due to the downgrade in my vision. I use it mainly to identify snail mail or to read a label. The Perkins Brailler is used to tag documents. If I skip this step, the item I failed to label in Braille is inevitably the one I need to find later. The process is time-consuming, but I enjoy substantial independence I wouldn't have otherwise.

"Victor Reader Stream" (my most recent acquisition) is an audible pocket-size device with internet connectivity. I can download podcasts, books, internet radio, and record personal memos. I put Braille labels on my basic mobile phone in order to find the keys. I can use voice dialing, but need help adding numbers to my contact list. Even with technology, I am still dependent on the help of sighted individuals. No one device, or even multiple devices, can replace the human eye, one of creation's wonders.

I continue to shake my head at the inappropriate responses of others. Approaching a window at the bank, I asked to cash a check. The teller turned to my friend and yelled, "How does she want it?" I felt like telling her, "I'm neither deaf nor dumb, just blind."

As I was on a mobility lesson, a man hollered at my instructor, "Tell her she's beautiful!" We were apparently hard of hearing. People sometimes feel the need to apologize for asking me if I *saw* something on TV. No need to change the lingo when talking to me. One day, a woman asked me the time. I flipped open my Braille watch and told her. She cooed, "Great job!" Would she have said that to a sighted person? Want to see something funny? Walk with me down a crowded street and watch my magical cane part the crowd, like Moses parting the Red Sea.

While working at Boylston College, I visited a store in town. Despite the cane in my hand, the cashier insisted on seeing my driver's license. The ID from the college wasn't good enough. Holding the cane higher didn't help either. I had to insist on speaking to the manager before I could complete my transaction. Common sense isn't so common after all. While still living in Jamaica, before the white cane, Grace and I were running to catch a bus. I accidentally bumped into a woman who harrumphed in disgust, "You blind or what?" We howled with laughter after apologizing. If she only knew!

Although I have by no means arrived, I have come a long way in learning to cope. Frustrations arise constantly, especially as my vision worsens, but I don't allow them to derail me. My disability is not an accident. God has given me a very strong reminder that I belong to Him. I am not immune to feelings of fear and insecurity, but I know where to turn when they come.

## I CAN LAUGH

That I can laugh is a very good thing,
And at myself, even better,
Or else I'd soon grow very thin
And die of high blood pressure.

## DIGITAL IMMIGRANT

Adaptive Technology is vast and intimidating.
I maneuver my way around this new country,
Moving with trepidation along its highways.
At the first cafe, a bountiful buffet awaits me.
My wallet groans; my neurons moan.
My senior brain resists but I persist.
Reluctantly, I select, then timidly ingest,
Recognizing this could be an antidote against Alzheimer's.

## MUSICAL JOY

My musical gifting came through Daddy, who played the mouth organ and loved to sing. He also played piano by ear. In 1970, we found a beautiful accordion in a pawn shop in Boston and purchased it for $70. It accompanied me through all my moves around the country, and has entertained many. Meanwhile, I had longed for a piano.

The year my spouse left, I decided to treat myself for Christmas. My apartment was too small for a full-sized piano, so I settled on an electronic keyboard. Pamela accompanied me to make the purchase. When she read the price tag, I cringed. I had never spent that kind of money on myself. Smiling, Pamela cajoled, "You deserve it! Get it!" Utilizing a promotional offer from my credit card, I purchased a Yamaha digital piano. The hours of pleasure this instrument provided for me, my children and many friends were priceless. Its therapeutic value could not be measured.

When the children left with their father on his visitation weekends, I felt an indescribable pain in my heart. I would sit at the keyboard, playing and singing until the pain was forgotten. Hours later, exhausted, I would sink into bed and sleep soundly. What an incredible gift God has given me in my ability to play by ear! The keyboard was 24 years old and sounding its age when I donated it and purchased a new, portable instrument. As I get older, it will be more difficult to handle the hefty accordion, but I hope to be playing the keyboard for a long time. This is one pleasure I will not be without.

I have been providing entertainment for the Christmas potluck at the gym and in the senior apartments where I now reside. I also play piano for the senior Sunday school class at church, and enjoy serving in convalescent ministry several times a month. I hear and feel the pleasure expressed by my audiences when I share old hymns and my original compositions. I sometimes write lyrics that fit a popular tune, as in the following song.

## CHRISTMAS JOY
(Tune: "Have Yourself a Merry Little Christmas")

Have yourself a very merry Christmas!
May your hearts be light!
Jesus Christ was born upon this holy night.
As you celebrate the Savior's birthday
Spreading joy around,
Let the people know true peace in Christ abounds.
He is not just a helpless babe
Born 2000 years ago.
He's the King who true freedom brings,
Yet so many in the world don't know.
Jesus died that we might be forgiven.
Spread this hope around.
Tell the world eternal life in Him is found,
And have yourself a very merry Christmas now!

One day Jesus will return from Heaven.
May your heart be right!
He will dry all tears and turn the dark to light.
He's the only one who can deliver
From the weight of sin.
Trust Him now and find deep-settled peace within.

Wars will cease, unity increase,
When He reigns as Prince of Peace.
Every knee then to Him will bow,
Come adore the Savior now.
Open up your heart, make room for Jesus,
Let the Savior in.
Find the true contentment that His presence brings,
And have yourself a very merry Christmas now! 2012


## GLAD TO BE ALIVE

Some women do not like to tell their age.
For me, each year is just another gauge
Of how much God has brought me through,
The blessings He each day renews.
I'm glad to be alive at 65!

My kids are grown and gone and doing well;
Me, I'm alive and kicking! Can't you tell?
Still useful though I'm growing old,
The wisdom gained is more than gold.
I'm glad to be alive at 65!

My hair is thinning and my joints they creak;
My back hurts when I'm too long on my feet.
I go to bed wearing Depends,
Insomnia is my new friend,
But I'm glad to be alive at 65!

There are things I can't remember and that's good;
Some people I forget, I really should.
If that's not you, just say your name;
I'll smile and say, "So glad you came!"
I'm glad to be alive at 65!

I do not know the things tomorrow holds,
But I know that my God is in control.
He's been with me for 65,
Through many snares, kept me alive.
I pray He'll grant another 25! 2013
(17-year cancer survivor)

"Blessed is the man who trusts in the Lord, whose confidence is in him. He is like a tree planted by the water...and never fails to bear fruit." Jeremiah 17:7, 8

## I TELL MY HEART THAT YOU LOVE ME

Flesh of my flesh I once nursed you
Nestled snug in my arms,
Singing songs softly to you,
Shielding you from all harm.
You are the son I once nurtured
Long before you could know
The way that laid before you,
The way you'd eventually go.

You are the son I have prayed for
And pray for still today,
That God would guard and guide you,
Direct your steps always.
I knew I was just a vessel
Used to fit you for life,
That one day I would release you
To the one who would be your wife.

Now you are grown and married,
And I'm so glad about that!
But I miss your hugs and your laughter
And long for just a chat.

I tell my heart that you love me,
But the weeks they come and go;
No card, no call, no email
Reassuring me that it's so.

My head says that you're busy
And I am busy too,
But my heart just knows I am missing
The closeness we once knew.
I tell my heart you still love me,
That you cannot really know
How much I long to see you,
So I try hard to let go.

I'm a sentimental woman
Who is getting on in years,
And missing the son I have succored
Moves me to shed these tears.
I'm just a mother who loves much,
Even with my faults and flaws,
And I need to be reminded
That you love me too, that's all.  2013

Avizi married Linda in the Redwood forest on February 7th, 2013. There was no family present, so I was naturally disappointed at first. Whatever his reason, a traditional wedding could have been awkward, given his complicated family ties. A few months later, I met Linda's parents, who visited California from Iowa. Their daughter is a precious and cherished complement to our family. We have stunning photographs of Avizi and Linda under the sequoias.

The young couple demonstrated their wisdom when they became debt-free a year after their union. Avizi works in the restaurant industry in a managerial position; Linda is a computer technician. They are both scuba divers, spending much of their free time under the sea, while I can't even stay afloat. Along with Agalia, they always spend time with me on my birthday and on Mother's Day.

Other times are up for grabs as they establish their own traditions and live their own lives, I suppose. I am still praying for God to send Agalia a husband, and I would love to see some grandchildren while I still can.

## REASSURING JOY

While working on this book, I was searching for a Scripture verse to complement the poem "Tomorrow," written during a tough year for my son and me. I selected Psalm 126:5, which promises joyful reaping after tearful labor. Still feeling a strain in our relationship, I kept praying. Just then, to my delight, an email from Avizi landed in my in-box. On reading it, I burst into tears of joy.

January 18, 2015

"Hello Mom,

Just wanted to tell you I Love You. I know we haven't had the best relationship and I haven't been around and you may feel I don't appreciate you, but I do. I really do. Because of you, I've become a successful man and I have an amazing life with a great career. You created my work ethic and drive. Without that I wouldn't be doing anything I am now. So thank you. Thank you very, very much. I love you.

Your son"

"I will praise you, O Lord, with all my heart; I will tell of all your wonders. I will be glad and rejoice in you; I will sing praise to your name, O Most High." Psalm 9:1, 2

# PART 15. CALM ASSURANCE

## *STORMY WEATHER*
(Tune: "I Know Who Holds Tomorrow")

In my flesh I am weak and mortal,
Plagued by many doubts and fears;
Pain and sickness have assailed me,
Deep heart-wounds bled many tears.
Near collapse beneath the burden,
My faltering spirit grasped God's hand.
From the shifting sand He drew me,
Placed me on a rock to stand.

Refrain:
Stormy weather unrelenting,
Howling winds just would not cease.
In that rock my Father hid me,
Whispering soothing words of peace.

Although the storm had made me tremble,
I heard that still small voice of peace;
Though still the distant thunders rumbled,
His voice from fear my heart released.
"Come, cast all your cares upon Me,
Bring your heavy burdens here;
For you, My grace will be sufficient;
I will drive away your fears.

In this world there is tribulation,
But, My child, do not despair.
Strength and courage I will give you
And I'm always with you here.
From this rock you'll gain perspective,
Understand My plans divine;
And no matter what assails you,
Just remember, you are Mine!" 2013

"For in the day of trouble he will keep me safe in his dwelling; he will hide me in the shelter of his tabernacle and set me high upon a rock." Psalm 27:5

## FAITH UNDER FIRE

In the midst of a trial, we don't always understand what God is doing and are fearful of the outcome. God knows we are only human; that is why He so often exhorts us to trust and not be afraid (Isaiah 12:2; 26:3; 35:3, 4; Luke 12:32). Our trust in God does not increase until we have walked through trials and experienced His presence, power and provision. He promised to walk with us through the storm, not around it.

The next test may be way bigger than any before, but, as a wise man said, "The task ahead of us is never as great as the power behind us." God will grant the needed faith, strength and endurance when the waters of life are the roughest, and the road I travel is the bumpiest. He will give me a song of joy and peace, even in the darkest night (Philippians 4:4-7).

A few weeks after I wrote the above paragraph, a new storm slammed into my harbor. Excruciating pain vibrated through my middle-section as another driver t-boned us on the passenger side. My caregiver was at the wheel. I was in the back on the passenger side. The car was totaled.

Crying and clutching my stomach, I immediately thought, "O God, there must be some internal damage!" I then thought of my nephew Jamal's upcoming wedding in Boston. The last time family had been together was for Faith's marriage to Winston, in 2007. A reunion was overdue so we all needed to be there. Unsure of the extent of my injuries, I worried about not making it.

Paramedics rushed me to the nearest ER. I was observed for a few hours, then dismissed with pain medication. The pain had subsided, so no X-ray or scan was done. I remained moderately stiff and sore until three days later. I awoke with a pounding headache and nausea; my right side was swollen; neck, arm, rib cage and breastbone pulsated with pain. The following Monday, an X-ray ruled out any broken ribs.

Ellen drove me to the airport on Wednesday, May 6th. Unable to lift even my purse without extreme discomfort, I was transported from curbside to plane in a wheelchair. While in Boston, I rested and the pain subsided. Jamal's marriage to Alexandra was held in a picturesque park, downtown Boston. All my siblings, as well as our children, were in attendance. There was much feasting and joviality. Returning home two weeks later, I assumed the effects of the accident were behind me.

A month after the collision, May 28th, I was sitting at the computer when a shock wave of pain jerked my shoulders. A surge of heat flooded my body and I became nauseated instantly. My whole torso was being crunched and twisted as if in a vise. Frantic, I stumbled to the telephone and sputtered my dilemma to the paramedics. The twisting and squeezing shifted to my chest. Thinking I was having a heart attack, I staggered to the bedroom and chewed two aspirins.

When paramedics arrived, I was vomiting violently between frenzied sobs. Spasms and vomiting were unrelenting for several hours after my stomach had been emptied of its contents. Despite medication, the spasms persisted. An EKG ruled out a heart attack. X-ray and CT scans were inconclusive.

Although the insurance company had accepted liability, several friends advised me to get a lawyer. Initially, I didn't think it necessary. A couple from church, who were chiropractors, agreed to treat me contingent on the insurance settlement. For the next several weeks, I received adjustments, deep-tissue massages and acupuncture, and was slowly improving. Experiencing some unpleasant side effects from the pain medication, I consulted my primary doctor. Without examining me, she decided that my problem was only musculoskeletal and refused my request to see a specialist.

One day mid-June, I called the insurance company and received contradictory information. Alarmed at the mounting medical bills, I hired a lawyer. He advised me to see an orthopedic specialist for a proper assessment. That same day, the apartment manager rang my doorbell with more frightful news. The neighbor had bedbugs and my apartment would have to be inspected.

Preparation for the inspection was a nightmare. I was in no shape for such an undertaking. Between crying, praying and calling friends, I began going from room to room, in stops and starts as my strength allowed. Over the next several days, friends and caregivers helped clear closets, bag clothing, food and toiletries, unscrew covers from electrical outlets, and move furniture away from the walls. I prayed fervently, "Lord, please don't let them find any bugs here!" Thank God, they didn't! A preventive spraying was nevertheless scheduled for July 1st.

Utterly fatigued and stressed, I was not eating well. I felt horrible and was losing weight rather rapidly. Something was very wrong. I called the doctor, insisting on seeing a specialist.

Breathing problems began as the bedbug fiasco ended. Assuming this was a side effect of the toxic spraying, I started using a rescue inhaler, though I hadn't needed one for years. The chiropractor expressed concern at my labored breathing and notified my primary doctor. On July 13th, still unable to get an appointment, I went to urgent care. Presuming my symptoms to be asthma, the attending physician administered a breathing treatment and prescribed Prednisone.

Nights were sheer torture as symptoms intensified. I tried to sleep sitting upright or bolstered by several pillows. When I dozed off, it was only to wake a few minutes later, gasping for air. My wild heartbeat and laborious breathing increased anxiety. The wheezing in my lungs sounded like a symphony. My tightening chest and a general feeling of foreboding added to the distress. I had no appetite and was weak from continued weight loss. The simplest task, like washing my face or walking across the room, left me panting as if I had just run a marathon.

More than two months after the accident, I saw the orthopedic specialist, who ordered three MRI's and prescribed Tramadol. Observing my heaving chest, he too showed concern.

"You need to go to the ER right away. I can arrange transportation for you right now." Noticing my reluctance, he made me promise to see my doctor that day, appointment or not; however, she was too busy to see me. As my condition steadily deteriorated that night, I called my medical helpline, hoping their advice would be different. It wasn't.

Gasping for air between sobs, I cried, "God, I can't do this!" I called Faith for support. She prayed with me and insisted I follow doctor's orders. Terrified of being hospitalized again, I didn't want to call the paramedics. Reluctantly, I called Ellen. We arrived at the ER by 5:30 the next morning.

An EKG and CT scan revealed fluid on my lungs. Several medications were administered intravenously and I was admitted. After an echo-cardiogram, the hospitalist delivered the bad news— congestive heart failure. I was stunned. What did this mean? Both my parents had congestive heart failure near the end of their lives, but I was only 67.

The hospitalist returned to my bedside with more disturbing news, "By the way, your kidney function is below normal. You are anemic. I will give you an injection of a drug called Epogen. It should help the anemia." Before this event, I had been taking just Benazapril for high blood pressure. I returned home with two additional prescriptions, Lasix (a water pill) and carvedilol (a beta-blocker).

My primary doctor was facing the computer, her back turned to me.

"I don't understand why you have anemia…unless there was some internal bleeding somewhere." She then mumbled something about me having kidney disease.

Aghast, I retorted, "You never ever told me there was a problem with my kidneys!" She waved at me dismissively, her back still to me, "Everybody knows everyone over a certain age has kidney disease!" I was dumbfounded!

I had been seeing this doctor for years and she had never even hinted at a problem with my kidneys. Although diabetic, I had kept my blood sugar under control with diet and exercise. Understanding kidney disease to be a late complication of advanced diabetes, I had given it no thought. At a friend's suggestion, I requested an angiogram. It would reveal any arterial blockages possibly contributing to the heart issues. The doctor's response was most unprofessional.

"I just need to know if I have any blockages," I replied in disbelief. She waved at me flippantly, "Of course you have blockages! Your cholesterol is high." Extremely disgruntled, I had blood work done and left her office.

The following week, at my request, a patient representative reviewed all my blood tests going back several years. On each one, the doctor's comments indicated that my kidneys were normal or stable. She never hinted at a need for concern. Now the latest test showed stage 3 kidney disease. I was done with that doctor!

The new PCP faced me as she listened to my concerns and answered my questions sensibly. She explained that my GFR (the measurement of kidney function) was 37; the normal is 90. I showed her my swollen tummy; she ordered a CT scan for the next morning. The scan detected an apparent tear in my aorta, the large artery descending from the heart. An emergency blood test showed my GFR at just 41, too low for a CT angiogram. The tear, I gathered, could have been caused by an injury or blow in a car accident, and could cause an arterial bleed-out. My head was spinning.

After a repeat echo-cardiogram, the cardiologist delivered a bombshell. I had severe mitral valve regurgitation and would need open heart surgery. He explained that, as blood was pumped from the heart, the mitral valves failed to close completely, allowing blood to flow backwards. This caused fluid buildup in the lungs and heart, resulting in congestive heart failure. He scheduled an angiogram for September 1st. Tears flowed as I listened. Was I in the twilight zone?

Fortunately, when I saw the nephrologist, the status of my kidneys had improved. It was safe to do the angiogram. There were no arterial blockages. Cholesterol was not an issue! The cardiologist decided to bypass open heart surgery and treat the mitral valve problem with increased medication. Great news!

Immobilized for several hours after the procedure, I was spoon-fed lunch by Agalia. "Mom," she giggled, "you're like a baby bird being fed by its mother." Talk about role reversal! I spent the night in the hospital due to fluid retention. The doctor doubled the dose of Lasix and added a potassium pill. His approach was to slowly increase the meds until normal breathing was restored. I was advised to consume a low-sodium diet, closely monitor fluid intake, and check my weight daily. Sudden weight gain of two pounds or more could indicate fluid retention.

The alleged aortic tear turned out to be a misdiagnosis, one less thing to worry about. Thank You, Jesus! Kidney function and blood pressure eventually stabilized, but breathing was still erratic. At the end of September, the cardiologist introduced the drug Aldactone. What a transformation! Within a week, I was breathing normally, my appetite was slowly returning, I resumed water aerobics, and was singing again. In four months I had lost 23 lbs. It was time for a wardrobe makeover.

My friend, Nichole, kept a wheelchair in her car. Walking was exhausting, so I used it quite often when she drove me to medical appointments. Her dad, Ed, who was 94 and also legally blind, sometimes accompanied us. Well, who do you suppose was pushing who in the wheelchair? You guessed it! The blind was pushing the blind and we managed to miss the ditch. We have chuckled often at that memory. Once I was breathing normally again, the whole experience seemed like a long night and a bad dream.

Thanks to my church family and friends whose prayers bolstered me through those worrisome days. Praise God, our awesome Creator! Our bodies are truly fearfully and wonderfully made. We too often take their functioning for granted. I am now a 20-year cancer survivor and a senior (68) with heart and kidney disease. Despite medical innovations and "age-defying" products, I know I will face the great equalizer at my appointed time (Job 14:5).

As I grow older, physical health will wane and storms will increase; nevertheless, God will always be faithful to walk with me through them. His trustworthy promise of ultimate deliverance and joy still stands.

"All men are like grass and all their glory like the flower of the field; the grass withers and the flower falls, but the word of the Lord stands forever." So, "Teach us to number our days a right, that we may gain a heart of wisdom." 1 Peter 1:24, 25; Psalm 90:12

## YOU CAN WEATHER THE STORM

You never know how you'll weather the storm
Until you find yourself in it,
But come they will those storms of life
With gale force winds of panic.
Your attitude as you ride out the storm
Can make you bitter or better.
You can decide to profit from pain
Or choose to wallow in it.

When your world falls apart, do not despair,
If in Jesus you have believed.
You can weather the storm, for the Lord will be there;
He'll show up at your point of need.
The lessons learned as you weather the storm
Will equip you to face your tomorrows,
To let others know that they too can be strong
And need not succumb to its sorrows. 2008

"Do not fear, for I am with you; do not be dismayed, for I am your God. I will strengthen you and help you..." Isaiah 41:10

## IS JESUS IN YOUR BOAT?

The perfect storm was raging
On the Sea of Galilee
While Jesus slept untroubled;
He is Master of the sea.

His disciples shook with terror,
Fearing burial in the deep;
Think of their consternation
Finding Jesus fast asleep.

"How can you sleep at this time?
Do you not care that we die?"
His answer was immediate:
"Peace, be still!" He cried.
As He rebuked the tempest
So He rebuked those fearful men.
Their "little faith" He chided;
They still did not know Him then.

Refrain:
Peace, be still! Peace, be still! Tell your soul it is well!
Peace, be still! Peace, be still! He is near, so all is well!

He will speak peace to your spirit
If He's in your boat, my friend;
Though the waters rise around you,
On His care you can depend.
His power is not diminished
By the power of the waves;
He loves you and has promised
To give courage and to save.

Take comfort in the knowledge
That whatever you go through,
However deep the waters,
Jesus will deliver you.
Though your circumstances tempt you
To lose courage and despair,
Just recall your *Ebenezers*
And remember He is near. 2013

(*Ebenezer* was a memorial stone erected by the Israelites to commemorate God's deliverance. 1 Samuel 7:7-12)

"Peace I leave with you; my peace I give you. I do not give to you as the world gives...In this world you will have trouble. But take heart! I have overcome the world." John 14:27; 16:33

# COMING ATTRACTIONS

God created me in His image to glorify and enjoy Him forever. His image in me has been marred by sin, yet even my fallen nature yearns for justice and peace in a troubled world. I have sinned, but God is completely holy and absolutely hates sin; it is an affront to His purity. Through Jesus, He has forgiven me. He will, in His time, eliminate everything that threatens my peace and joy. This guaranteed deliverance, procured by the death and resurrection of Jesus, is for all who acknowledge their flawed humanity and need for a Savior.

Human depravity, as expressed in the devaluing of life from the womb to the tomb, often rattles my faith. Murder of unborn babies; infants discarded in dumpsters; exploitation of children, women, the poor, disabled and elderly; infidelity and divorce; racism, gun violence, terrorism, and even my private rebellion against God's rules, are examples of evil that a Holy God will eliminate. He has promised to judge all unrepentant sinners. Hope and joy are rekindled when I remember that all evil will be eradicated at the return of Jesus, the one who died and is alive, holding the keys to death and hell; the Sovereign King and Judge of all the earth; the source of my joy.

To those who trust Him, He promises forgiveness and enduring freedom from sin and its consequences, a new world where peace and joy will flourish.

Jesus said: "Now is your time of grief, but I will see you again and you will rejoice, and no one will take away your joy...Do not let your heart be troubled; trust in God; trust also in me. In my Father's house are many rooms...I am going there to prepare a place for you...I will come back and take you to be with me...I have told you this so that my joy may be in you and that your joy may be complete." (Excerpted from John 14-16.) It is towards this ultimate fulfillment of joy that I journey. Will you come with me to my Father's house?

## BRIGHT NEW WORLD
(Tune: White Christmas)

I'm dreaming of a bright new world
Just like the one the Lord first made,
Where creation's wonder is unencumbered
By sin, suffering, or pain.
I'm dreaming of a world where children
Will play with lions as with lambs,
Where Jesus Christ will be the light,
When all that's wrong will be made right.

I'm dreaming of a new creation,
Where Jesus Christ will reign as King.
There'll be no injustice, no need for hospice,
For we will live eternally.
I'm dreaming of a heavenly body
No longer plagued by pain and death.
God Himself will wipe away all tears,
And forever there'll be no night there.

I am dreaming of that glorious morning
When I shall see my Savior's face;
Just to look upon Him, just one smile from Him
Will all the cares of earth erase.
I'm dreaming of a Heavenly choir,
Of harmony earth never knew,
When from every nation, tribe and tongue,
We will worship God with a new song.

"The ransomed of the Lord...will enter Zion with singing; everlasting joy will crown their heads. Gladness and joy will overtake them, and sorrow and sighing will flee away." Isaiah 51:11

## *YOUR KINGDOM COME*

There is so much heartache and despair this side of Heaven,
But Jesus said that one day very soon He will appear.
With divine authority He'll consummate His kingdom
And all earth's terrors then will disappear.

Our Father promises to wipe all tears from our eyes,
For where the King of Kings resides sin's sting cannot remain.
Christ, the Faithful and the True, will banish every evil
And in His kingdom joy and peace will reign.

Quickly come, Lord Jesus, and remove us from this darkness
To that glorious city where Your light forever shines.
May Your kingdom come, Your will be done in all creation!
May all the joy You promise soon be mine.

O to see the nail prints that You bore for my redemption
When on Calvary's cross You paid the ransom for my sin!
Of Your grace and mercy, love and justice, wrath and splendor,
With saints and angels I'll forever sing.

"For the Lamb...will be their shepherd; he will lead them to springs of living water. And God will wipe away every tear from their eyes...There will be no more death or mourning or crying or pain, for the old order of things has passed away." Revelation 7:17; 21:4

## WE SHALL BE LIKE JESUS

When our glorious King appears, we shall be like Jesus.
When we meet Him in the air, we shall be like Jesus.
Unity will be preserved, we will love without reserve
Even those who've wounded us, for we'll be like Jesus.

There will be no sin in us when we are with Jesus.
We'll be dressed in righteousness, all adorned by Jesus.
Pride, rebellion, selfishness, envy, malice, bitterness
Will no longer be our dress when we're clothed like Jesus.

What a joyful happy day when we all see Jesus.
Sin's desires gone away, we shall be like Jesus.
We will join the heavenly band singing praises to the Lamb,
Worshipping the great "I Am" who makes us like Jesus.

"...there is rejoicing in the presence of the angels of God over one sinner who repents." Luke 15:10

"To him who is able to keep you from falling and to present you before his glorious presence without fault and with great joy—to the only God, our Savior be glory, majesty, power and authority through Jesus Christ our Lord..." Jude 1:24, 25

# FAMILY ALBUM

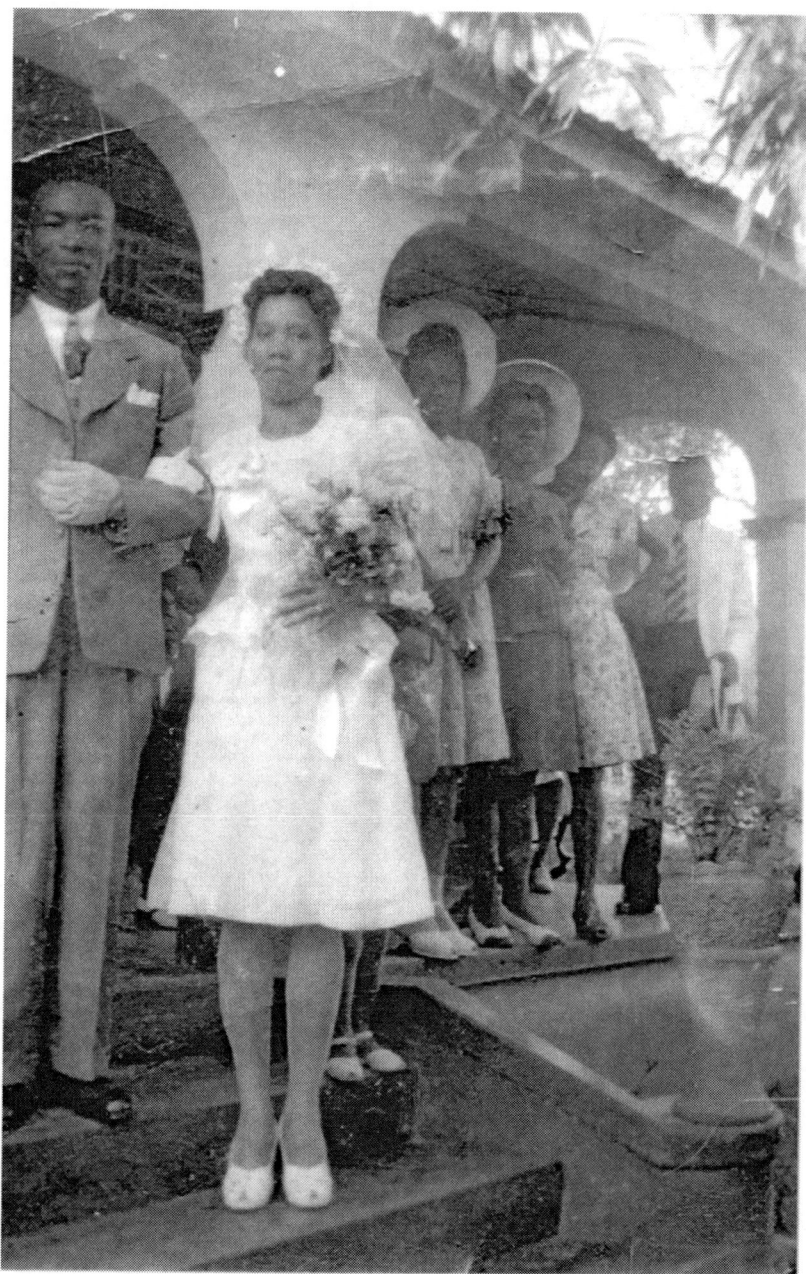

**Daddy and Mama Creating a Covenant - 1947**

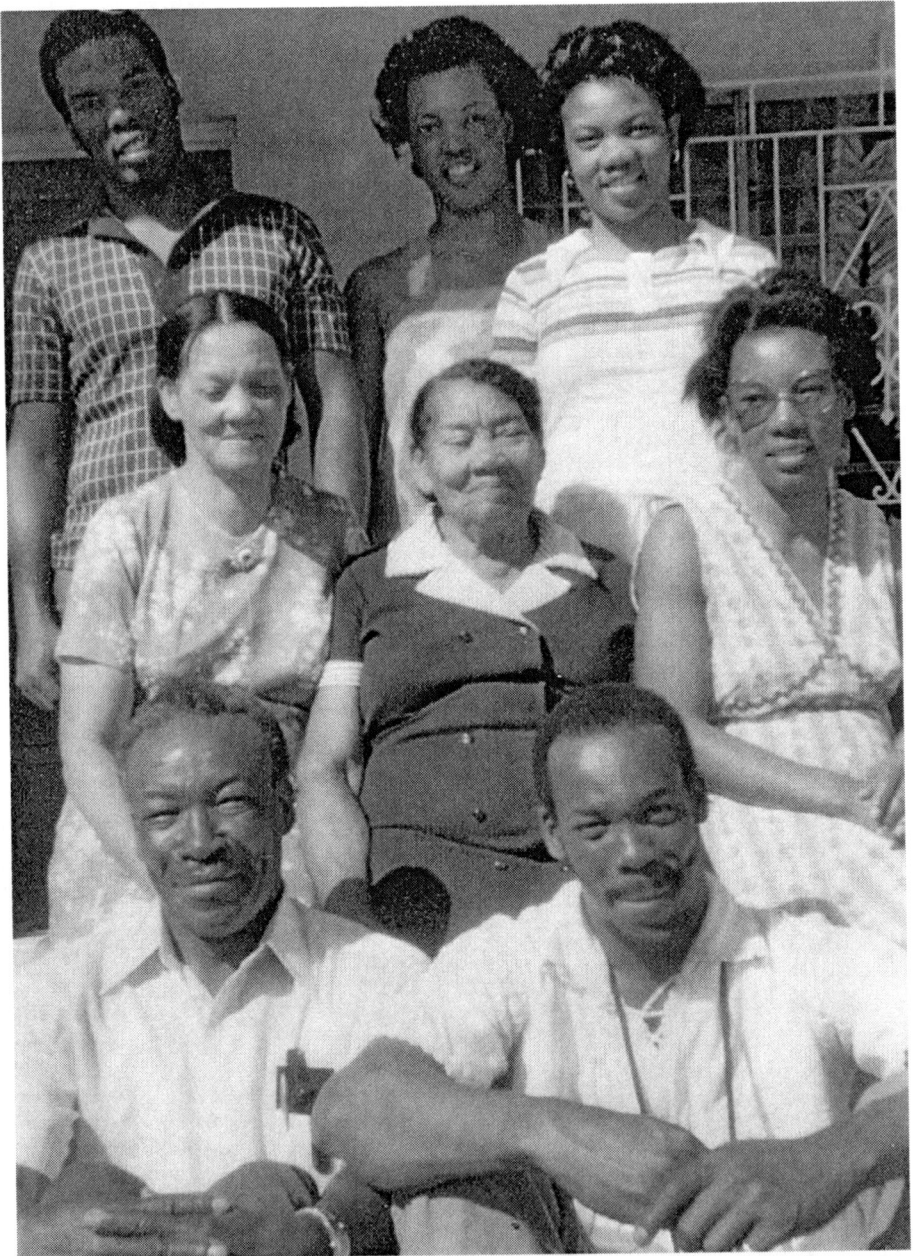

**Joy's Family of Origin "Less Two" - 1977**

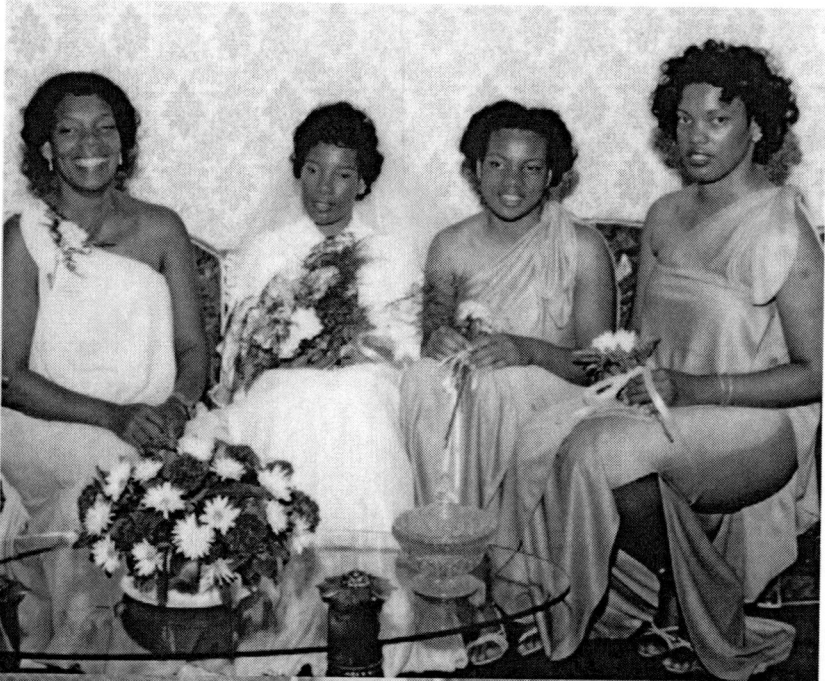

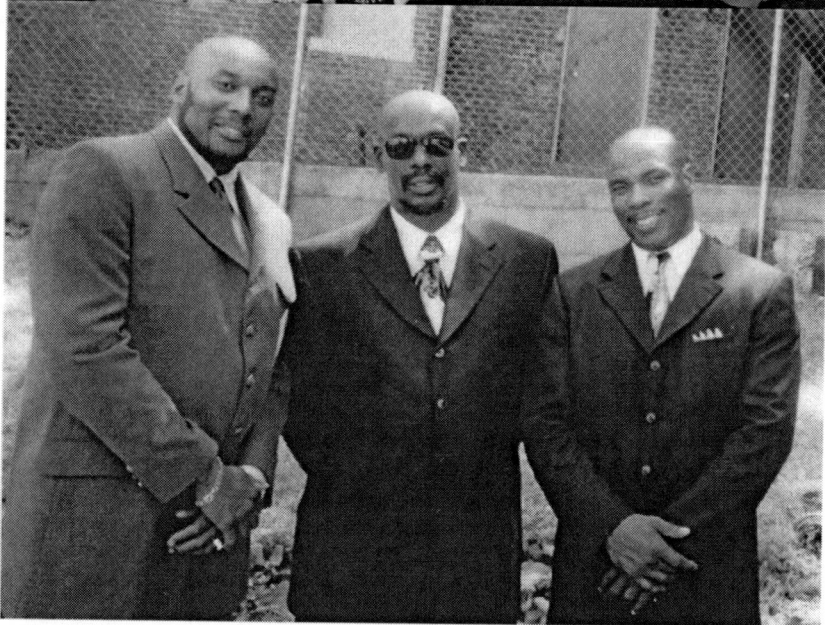

**Joy and Siblings**

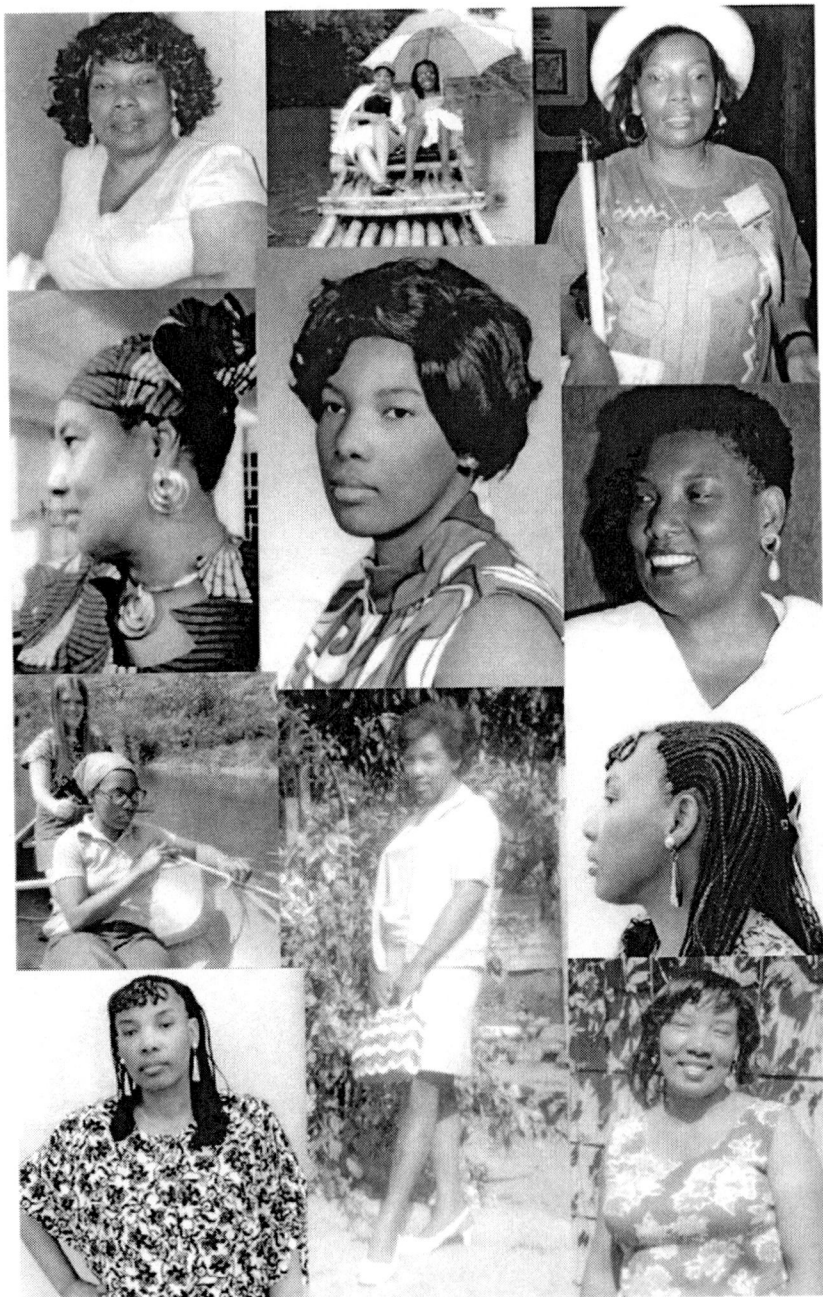

**Faces of Joy**

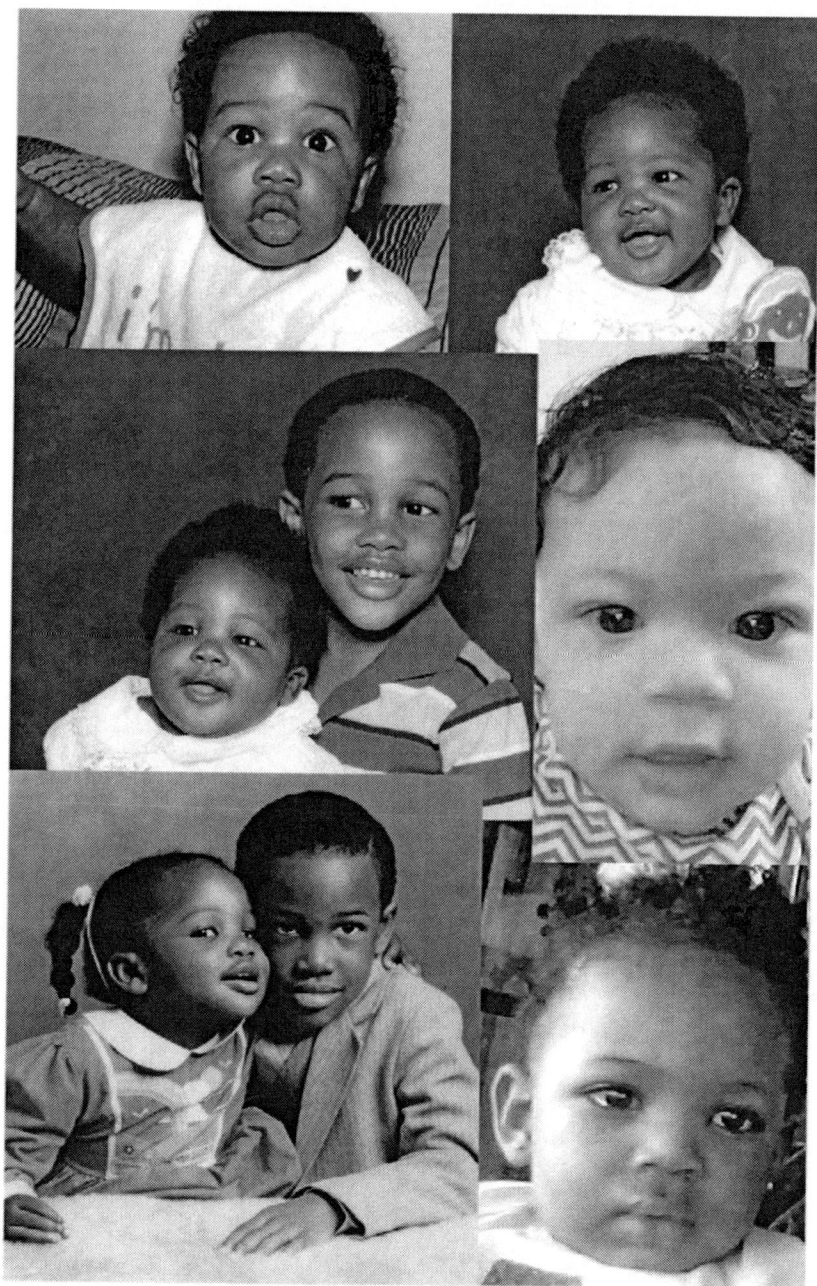

**Joy's Babies with Cousins
Olivia J. and Olivia F.**

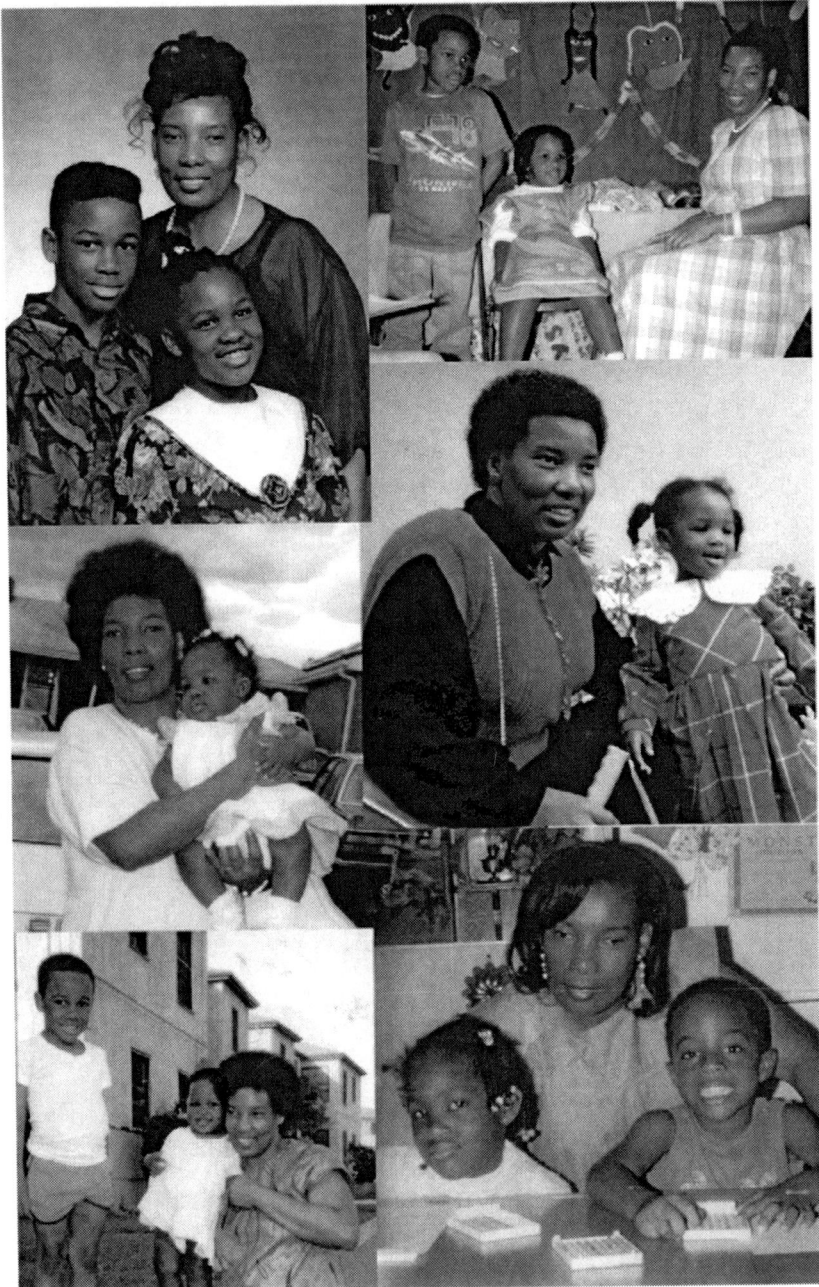

**Joy and Children**

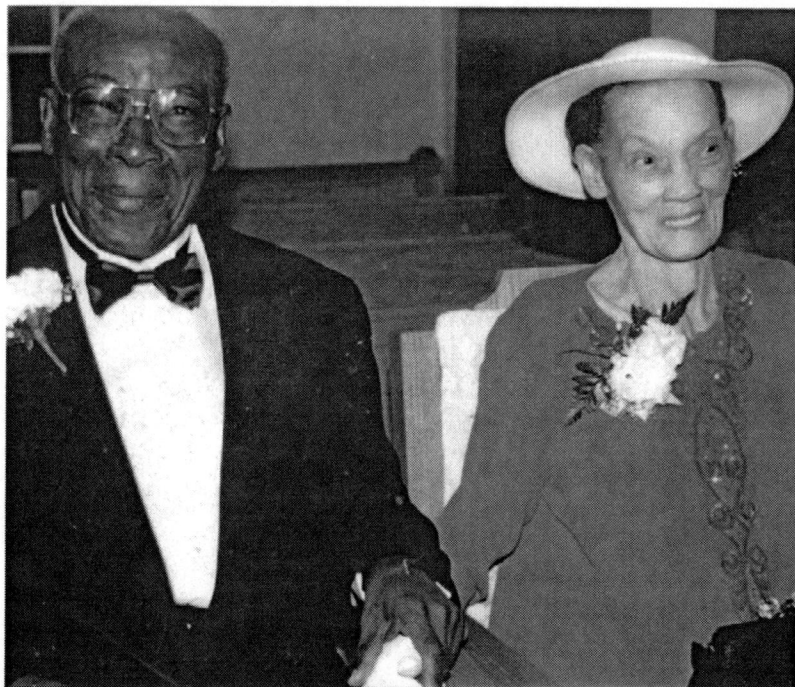

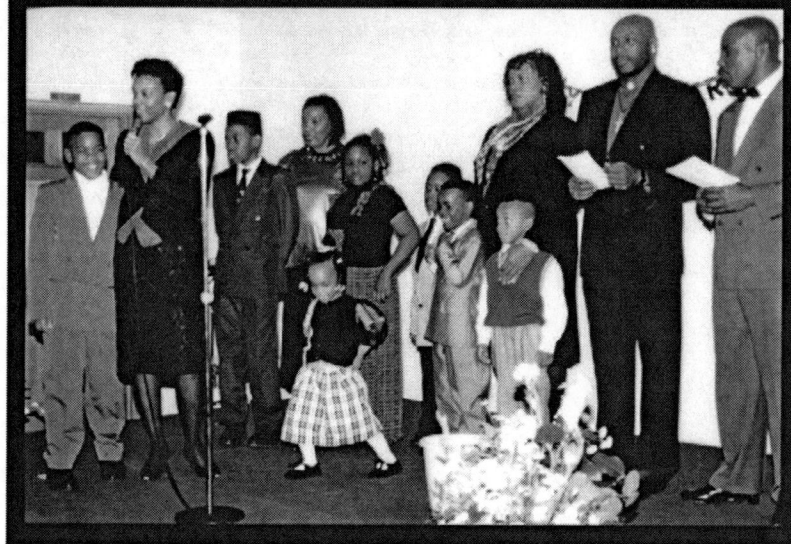

**Celebrating Their Covenant - 1995**

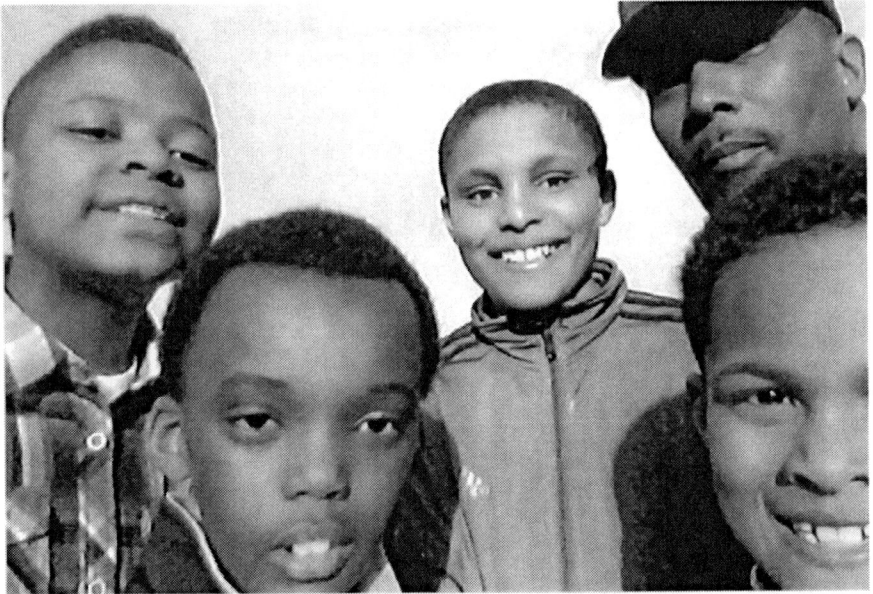

**Danny's Clan**

# MORE ABOUT THE AUTHOR

Just before submitting this book for publication, I received wonderful news. Fifteen months after the diagnosis of congestive heart failure, my heart is back to its normal size and all the valves are closing completely. I am thankful to God for His watch care, for Dr. David Yang, my diligent cardiologist, and for all my praying friends.

As a 20-year cancer survivor, I continue to be an advocate and speaker for various organizations, using my gifts of poetry and music to encourage others. Following is a select list of venues where I have been published and/or have appeared as Guest Poet/Musician/ Survivor Speaker:

The Wellness Community, Pasadena, CA, Newsletter, April 1998
Black Women's Health Task Force, Pasadena, CA, 1999
American Cancer Society, Personal Advocacy Workshop, 1999
City of Hope, Duarte, CA, Hope Notes, Feb/March 2003
The Wellness Community, Silver Saturday, 2005
Miller's River Senior Center, Cambridge, MA, 2006
South Pasadena Review, 4/25/2007
Relay for Life, South Pasadena, CA, 2007, 2008
Cruise For the Cure, Inflammatory Breast Cancer Foundation, 2008
"Pink" Day...Survivors' Forum, County of Los Angeles, Department of Ombudsman, 2008
"Increasing the Voice of African Americans in Breast Cancer Research," City of Hope, 2010
"Elevate Your Game," Compton High School, Compton, CA, 2011
Cancer Minority Awareness Forum, City of Hope, 2011-2016
Broadway Health Center, San Gabriel, CA, 1992-2016
Alderwood Manor Convalescent Hospital, San Gabriel, CA, 2012-2016
Sunrise Senior Living, San Marino, CA, 2013-2014
Khemobuddy, Annual Luncheon, Pasadena, CA, 2015
Vessels of Hope, Pasadena, CA, 2015
Atherton Baptist Homes, Alhambra, CA, 2015
*Writing For Wellness: A Prescription for Healing*, coauthor with Julie Davey, 2007
"Visions of Wellness," http://www.writingforwellness.com, 2010

CPSIA information can be obtained
at www.ICGtesting.com
Printed in the USA
FSOW02n1116020517
33790FS

9 781634 917438